The Official
Snack
Guide
for Beleaguered
Sports Parents

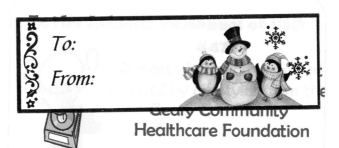

To:

From:

Geary Community
Healthcare Foundation

The Official Snack Guide

for Beleaguered Sports Parents

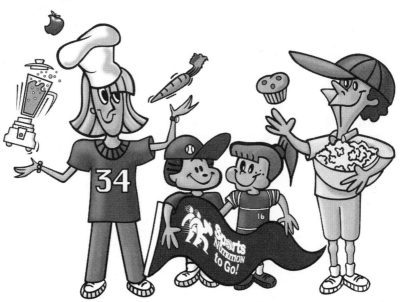

Dawn Weatherwax, RD, LD, ATC/L, CSCS
Rita Nader Heikenfeld, CCP
Joan MacEachen Manzo, RN, BSN
and Ellen Shuman

WellCentered Books
Cincinnati, Ohio

The Official Snack Guide for Beleaguered Sports Parents
By Dawn Weatherwax, RD, LD, ATC/L, CSCS, Rita Nader Heikenfeld, CCP,
Joan MacEachen Manzo, RN, BSN, and Ellen Shuman

Library of Congress Control Number   2001   130176
ISBN   0-9702831-0-5

Book Designed by Chad Planner and Eliza Tassian

Sports Nutrition To Go!
WellCentered Books
3414 Edwards Rd.
Cincinnati, OH 45208

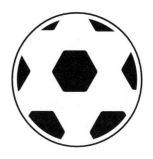

Acknowledgments

To all of you who were appropriately amused when we first shared our idea for this book…your enthusiasm and encouragement were greatly appreciated! Please accept our heartfelt thanks, along with your long-awaited copy of this book.

Also, a special "Thank You" to Kroger for providing the fine foods used in the testing of our recipes.

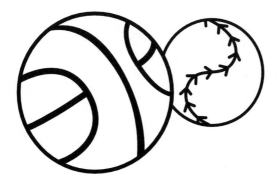

Table Of Contents

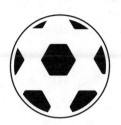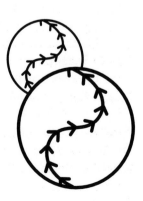

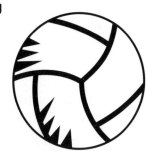
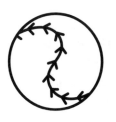

Welcome

To The Official Snack Guide For Beleaguered Sports Parents

A Sports Nutrition guide and snack book for sports parents? You bet! This book was conceived and written by a child-friendly team of colleagues, all of whom are affiliated with a Sports Nutrition practice called Sports Nutrition To Go!. Two of us are parents. All four of us have active kids in our lives. You name it, our children play it.

Our growing children, like yours, require good nutrition. And, most enthusiastically, they demand and deserve "cool" snacks!

Yes, our children have informed us that snacking should be "fun"! As conscientious, and sometimes anxiety-driven parents, we also believe snacks should have some identifiable nutritional value. But when we went looking for user-friendly Sports Nutrition information (written so Moms and Dads could take it and run), and for corresponding foods our children would actually eat, we came up very, very short.

And that's how this book came to be. We saw a need and a potential win. We knew we could come up with healthy snack options our children would like. With idea in hand, we cooked up *The Official Snack Guide For Beleaguered Sports Parents* and we had a blast!

This is who we are and how we came to be a working team...

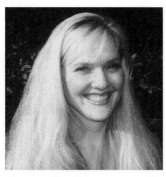

Dawn Weatherwax, RD, LD, ATC/L, CSCS

Dawn Weatherwax, our Sports Nutrition expert, is a Nebraska Corn Husker from way back. Dawn is a registered dietitian, an athletic trainer, and a certified strength and conditioning specialist. She's the nutrition expert behind our Sports Nutrition To Go! consulting business. In addition to her work with individual athletes, and her group presentations to high school and college coaches, Dawn consults with several Olympic athletes and pro teams in Cincinnati, including the Cincinnati Reds. To learn more about Dawn and her services, please visit our website, **www.SportsNutritionToGo.com**

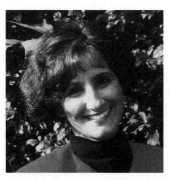

Rita Nader Heikenfeld, CCP

Certified Culinary Professional Rita Nader Heikenfeld is a well-known cooking teacher, award winning syndicated food columnist, and media personality in Cincinnati. She's best known for creating healthy, low fat recipes that appeal to the whole family. Rita's true interest in Sports Nutrition began very close to home. Her sons Jason and Shane are both competitive runners. Sometimes in the past, when her boys competed at full-speed, they experienced exhaustion and were plagued by muscle cramps. In an effort to learn as much as possible about how to keep her own sons healthy, Rita quickly discovered that reliable Sports Nutrition advice was not easy to find. Then she met Sports Nutritionist Dawn Weatherwax. You know what they say about necessity being the "mother of invention". Well, this mother took a great idea and ran with it! And that's how this book began to take shape.

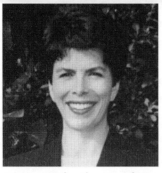

Joan MacEachen Manzo, RN, BSN

Joan MacEachen Manzo is a registered nurse and currently works as a physician liaison for a major health care system. She's the mother of a toddler named Isabella and a fourth grade basketball player named Annamarie. (Annamarie tested all the recipes found in this book. If Annamarie liked it, it made the cut.) Joanie comes from a long line of restaurateurs, and has operated a cooking-to-go business that prepared and delivered pre-cooked meals to busy working parents. Joanie is a cook extraordinaire! In certain circles she is well known (legendary actually) for her casual dinner parties where everyone sits around her coffee table feasting on her latest culinary "experiments". Being one of her friends definitely has its perks!

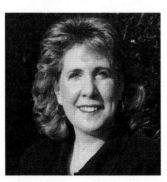

Ellen Shuman

Ellen Shuman is one of Joanie's friends. Ellen is the person who gathered and mixed all the ingredients and creative people needed to make this *Official Snack Guide*. Ellen is the founder and Executive Director of WellCentered, Inc., the parent corporation of the Hyde Park Wellness Center, Sports Nutrition To Go!, the Acoria Eating Disorders Treatment Center, and A WEIGH OUT; An End To Diets and

Out-of-Control Eating (www.aweighout.com). Dawn and Ellen are partners in Sports Nutrition To Go! and Rita and Joanie have presented many cooking classes at Ellen's Wellness Center. As a former Peabody and Emmy Award winning broadcast journalist, Ellen was just the right person to serve as this book's chief "cook".

That's who we are. Here's what we have to offer.
Inside our *Official Snack Guide* you'll find general nutrition guidelines for children, as well as an introduction to the basic tenets of Sports Nutrition. Please utilize the Sports Nutrition information to whatever degree it is relevant to your children's lives.

Please take full advantage of our recipes because they're all simple to make...and because they taste really good!

With the hope that this *Official Snack Guide* will encourage parents and children to play together in the kitchen as well as on the field, we designed many of our recipes with young helpers in mind. So roll up the sleeves of your children's jerseys...and have a ball!

QUESTIONS? COMMENTS?
If you'd like to contact any of the authors of this book, call (513)321-7202, email info@SportsNutritionToGo.com, or write to Sports Nutrition To Go!, 3414 Edwards Rd., Cincinnati, OH 45208.

TO ORDER ADDITIONAL BOOKS
You'll find an Order Form on page 177. To order directly from our website, visit SportsNutritionToGo.com and click Official Snack Guide, or call (513)321-7202, or our toll-free number, 1-866-GO SNACK.

ATTENTION ORGANIZATIONS AND SCHOOLS
For fundraising and educational purposes, quantity discounts are available on bulk purchases of this book. For more information contact WellCentered Books, (513)321-7202, info@SportsNutritionToGo.com.

Chapter One

Sports Nutrition To Go!

One morning you wake up and it has happened. You find yourself thrown into a world for which you have no training. Today, you are a Soccer Mom or a Basketball Dad. And it's your turn to bring a snack. The pressure is on.

"High drama is in", says an amused and tired soccer Mom named Mary Beth Smith. If a snack doesn't "gush, morph or implode", Mary Beth fears she will fail miserably in her daughter Tara's eyes. The word is out in their neighborhood. Orange slices just don't cut it anymore.

Ann Shuman says "guilt" is her predominant emotion. When it comes to planning snacks, this working mother of three says she waffles between "doing the right thing" and buying her children all the junk food she loved when she was a child. In case this news hasn't reached your town yet, Twinkies and HoHos are not considered "PC" anymore.

Ken Matthew says he often had to hold his breath and count to ten when it was his turn to drive daughter Britt's carpool. Without fail, they'd be running late. Then, just seconds from the field, Britt would yell from the backseat, "Hey Dad, I forgot to tell you. It's our turn to bring the team snacks". Ken learned that once you take on the role of sports parent, with all associated responsibilities, there's no turning back!

Then there are the important "gastronomic" concerns that every parent faces. If your child's kick-off time is at nine in the morning, do you feed him a big breakfast and risk an upset stomach on the sideline...or do you offer a light breakfast and risk energy drain mid-event? And how do you know how much fluid your daughter should drink, before, during, and after a game, to reduce the likelihood of dehydration or injury?

With these real life questions in mind, *The Official Snack Guide For Beleaguered Sports Parents* offers practical, easy to implement suggestions and strategies. We want you and your child to have the home field advantage. So, our Sports Nutrition recommendations for "game day" are designed to improve your child's concentration, reduce fatigue and injuries, and avoid upset tummies.

You won't find any "pie in the sky" recommendations in this Guide. As busy parents, we know better! Instead, you'll find useful lists like "Grocery Store Pick-Ups On the Run". In Chapter Five, you'll learn how to "Score Points In The Drive-Through Lane". Before you reach our recipe chapters, Seven through Eleven, we'll answer many questions commonly asked by Moms, Dads, Grandparents, and Coaches who care about the nutritional needs of an active child.

Your options for using this book are as follows. Read all about the basics of Sports Nutrition and hydration, and how to apply these simple suggestions to your child athlete. Or simply punt and pass all of the nutrition facts and go right for the recipes! We promise our recipes will taste just as good, with or without the nutrition lesson.

The referee just blew her whistle. Our first quarter begins now.

Chapter Two

Sports Nutrition Playbook For Parents

The Best Kept Secret

At any level of competition, Olympic or Little League, it has long been common knowledge that athletes can improve performance through a winning combination of practice, mental focus and physical conditioning.

Now there's something new, something very exciting. Today we offer new strategies for maximizing concentration, minimizing fatigue and reducing susceptibility to injury. We're talking about the best-kept secret in the world of sports: Sports Nutrition.

Top athletic coaches all over the world are becoming aware of Sports Nutrition as a powerful tool for both injury prevention and performance enhancement. Sports Nutrition strategies are effective, easy, and inexpensive to implement.

As with any expert advice, the Sports Nutrition guidelines outlined here should be applied appropriately. For example, if your child is the average active child playing on neighborhood and school teams, attention to an overall healthy diet, adequate fluid intake, and food choices on game day are likely all that your child needs.

On the other hand, if your son or daughter is a serious competitor, maybe vying for a college sports scholarship or an Olympic Gold Medal, then attention to other Sports Nutrition tools may also be of value, i.e., pre-event and post-event meal planning, daily training menus, lean muscle mass to body fat ratio, etc. (For that kind of specialized planning, we recommend consultation with a registered dietitian with expertise in Sports Nutrition. We invite you to visit our website, SportsNutritionToGo.com for more information about our consulting services.)

That said…The general nutrition and Sports Nutrition information that follow are designed for any and all growing, active children. Our Playbook For Parents begins here.

What Every Parent Should Know About Fluids

Do you know if your child is currently drinking enough fluid before, during, and after a practice or game?

Here's Why Fluid Intake Is So Important
• Proper hydration is especially important for children because a child's body takes longer to adjust to heat and humidity than does an adult's. Also, children produce more body heat and don't sweat as much as adults do at the same exertion level. So in hot weather a young athlete is at increased risk for dehydration
• In the body, water works as a shock absorber. If water is deficient, even for a brief period of time, there's less fluid present to protect the joints. This can make a young athlete more prone to injury

- Every 2.2 lbs of water lost during exertion results in the following:
  1. Heart rate increases eight beats per minute—with an elevated heart rate the body has to exert more energy to do the same job
  2. Decline in cardiac oxygen output—this means less oxygen is going to the person's muscles which can lead to a decrease in athletic performance
  3. Core temperature rises from 98.6 to 99.14 Fahrenheit—when the body experiences this rise in temperature it has to work harder to cool down. In an effort to cool down, the body pulls fluids away from the working muscles and redistributes the fluids to vital organs. Since muscular movement is dependent on the presence of water, low concentrations of water in the muscles can cause muscle weakness, muscle cramping, and loss of the critical control needed by an athlete for peak performance
- Athletic performance can decline as much as 10% with as little as 1% body fluid loss, i.e., a 100 lb. athlete has to lose only 1 lb. of body fluid for a 10% performance decline to occur

Fluids We Recommend

1. Cold Water

Research shows water is best absorbed by the body when it is consumed at approximately 40 degrees Fahrenheit. That's refrigerator temperature. That's a fact we find interesting, but not necessarily critical to the successful hydration of your child. How cold the water may be is most relevant for this reason. A child is more likely to drink the water if it is cool rather than warm. So we recommend an insulated water bottle, or use of a lot of ice in a non-insulated one.

The ice will melt throughout the event, guaranteeing enough cool water to last the length of the event.

2. Diluted Fruit Juice or Fruit Drink

Diluting fruit juice is an inexpensive way to create your own sports drink. Reduced with water to a 6-8% carbohydrate solution, diluted fruit juice will efficiently deliver just the right amount of carbohydrates to working muscles. (See page 29 to learn more about the important role carbohydrates play in muscle performance and injury prevention.)

Why dilute the juice? Non-diluted, the fruit juice has twice the concentration of carbohydrates as a diluted one. That means it will take longer to digest. Fruit juice sitting in your child's stomach may increase the chances of an upset stomach at the very height of activity. The diluted drink will taste weak. But it will still do what you want it to: hydrate your child and provide the necessary energy for intense play.

To dilute a powdered juice drink like lemonade in a packet, or any juice from concentrate, always use at least twice the water recommended on the package.

Tip Always choose a fruit juice or fruit drink that contains 100% of the recommended daily value of Vitamin C. This ensures that your child is drinking a beverage with some nutritional value vs. a drink with only empty calories.

3. Sports Drinks

Sports drinks typically contain a 6-8% carbohydrate solution, making them easily digestible and a quick source of energy. They come in cool colors and kids think they're fun to drink. Very young athletes, who may not tolerate the taste of a diluted fruit juice, may be more likely to drink a sports drink. Advantage, Mom! The disadvantage is this. Sports drinks cost more than water, and sometimes more than juice, so weigh the pros and cons. Examples of sports drinks include, Gatorade, POWERaDE, ALL SPORT, etc.

When To Offer Water vs. Juice vs. a Sports Drink

Prevailing wisdom indicates cold water is just fine if the activity lasts less than 60 minutes.

If an activity lasts 60 to 90 minutes, or longer, a 6-8% carbohydrate sports drink or diluted fruit juice (to 6-8% carbs) is recommended.

How Much Fluid Is Enough?
General Guidelines For Fluid Intake

- The day of a game your child should be drinking water throughout the day
- 2 to 3 hours before your child leaves for an event your child should drink at least one 8-16 oz glass of water or fruit juice (non-diluted is OK if the event is at least one hour away from its start time), or a sports drink
- Just before you head out the door, fill a 32 oz water bottle. Encourage your young athlete to drink at least a fourth of it, 8 oz, on the way to the event

If you get a transparent water bottle with measurements down the side, you can get permanent markers and make colorful indicators your child can use to figure out how much to drink and when.

Tip

- As your child is warming up, encourage him to drink another fourth of the water (to the next colored line)—making that a total of 16 oz or 2 cups drunk since leaving the house
- Teach your child how important it is to drink a few ounces from the water bottle every chance he gets once the game begins—even to the point of over drinking. Educate your child that thirst is not a good indicator of hydration. By the time a child is thirsty, he is already somewhat dehydrated
- Ideally, half way through the event your child should finish off another 8 oz, for a total of 24 oz drunk since leaving the house
- By the end of the event, the bottle should be empty, 32 oz of liquid consumed
- Right after the game, refill the water bottle for after-the-game hydration and encourage the child to drink as much as he or she wants. (Remember to explain to the child why it's important to replenish lost fluids.)

> In really hot weather, we also encourage use of a spray bottle with water in it. Throughout the game the young athlete can mist himself/herself. This will help the child's body better regulate temperature.
>
> **Tip**

Other Ways To Tell If Your Child Is Drinking Enough

A simple way to gauge if a child is getting enough fluids during athletic endeavors is through urine output. If your child urinates every one to two hours and her urine is light yellow rather than dark, and plentiful rather than concentrated, she's getting enough fluid.

Of course the downside of drinking plenty of fluids during a sporting event is the potential need for bathroom breaks. But that's OK. There are bathroom facilities at most playing fields. And the upside greatly outweighs the down-side. Your child will be well-hydrated and healthy, and will play his or her very best.

The general guidelines we just outlined are more than adequate for most active children. But if your child is partic-ipating in intense competition, where he or she is likely to experience significant fluid loss and potential muscle strain, you may want to experiment with this next formula. This is an easy way to calculate exact fluid loss and fluid replace-ment needs.

Formula For Determining A "Serious" Athlete's Optimal Fluid Needs

To achieve peak performance, the goal is to consistently replace any fluids an athlete is likely to lose.

- 2-3 hours before a workout or competition, the athlete should drink 2 cups, 16 oz of fluids
- Then, 1 hour before a workout or competition, the ath-lete should drink 1 cup, 8 oz of fluid
- 15 minutes before the workout or competition, the ath-lete drinks ½ cup, 4 oz of fluid
- Immediately before the workout or competition, weigh and record the athlete's weight
- Every 10-20 minutes during the workout or competition the athlete should drink ½ cup, 4 oz of fluid
- Then, right after a workout or competition, weigh the athlete. Then have the athlete drink 3 cups, 24 oz of fluid for every pound of weight lost
- Experiment with this formula and then adjust accordingly for each different athletic activity, until the athlete's weight remains the same from the start of the activity through to the very end

Please Note... There may be some additional adjustments needed when playing in particularly hot weather.

Pickle Juice
For Muscle Cramps?

Tip

That's what the Trainers at the University of Northern Iowa use to treat muscle cramps. According to Darryl Conway, UNI's Director of Sports Medicine, when all other prevention techniques fail such as hydration, good nutrition, conditioning and stretching, pickle juice works as a treatment for chronic muscle cramps. Conway says when his college athletes drink 2 oz of sweet or dill pickle juice 10 minutes before exercising, even the most chronic crampers remain cramp-free during high intensity exercise. His trainers have found that 2 oz of straight apple cider vinegar works well, too. (Some trainers use mustard.) But pickle juice appears to be the most palatable. The obvious common ingredient here is vinegar. But, to date, there is no research that explains the mechanism by which this treatment works. Conway says, if a trainer wanted to try this remedy on a younger athlete who suffers from chronic muscle cramps, he'd suggest cutting the amount of pickle juice down to a capful, about 1 oz. See what happens.

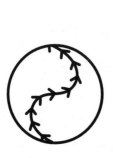

Tip

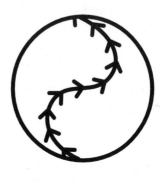

Nutrition 101:
The Home Field Advantage

A Balanced Diet For Your Active Children

They're active and they're growing! That means your children's nutritional needs are greater now than they will be at any other time in their lives. Now is the time to ensure that your children are getting all the nutrients needed for optimal growth.

Daily intake for all healthy children over two years of age should emphasize the eating of complex carbohydrates and moderate amounts of fat and protein; enough to support both growth and your child's level of physical activity. Your child's daily nutrition breakdown should look something like this: 55-60% Carbohydrates, 12-15% Protein, 30% Fat.

How do you ensure a balanced diet when children today think the names of the food groups are "Frozen, Fast, Take-Out, and Nuke-able"? We heard it from our parents and from our health teachers, and it's still the best advice. Eat the recommended daily servings from every food group: Grains, Vegetables, Fruits, Dairy, and Meat.

On the next two pages you'll find the USDA's (U.S. Department of Agriculture's) two Food Guide Pyramids. In 1999, the USDA came out with new guidelines designed specifically for children ages 2-6. If you follow the Food Guide's servings recommendations and provide healthy food choices, your child should get the appropriate number of calories and the *Recommended Daily Allowances of important nutrients each day. (We've listed sample serving sizes, too.)

SOURCES
* *Recommended Daily Allowances,* 10th Revised Edition, National Academy of Sciences, National Academy Press, Washington D.C.
* *Food Finder; Vitamin & Mineral Source Guide,* Fourth Edition, ESHA Research, Salem, OR, 1995

Food Guide Pyramid

Ages 2 to 6

Approximately 1600 calories a day

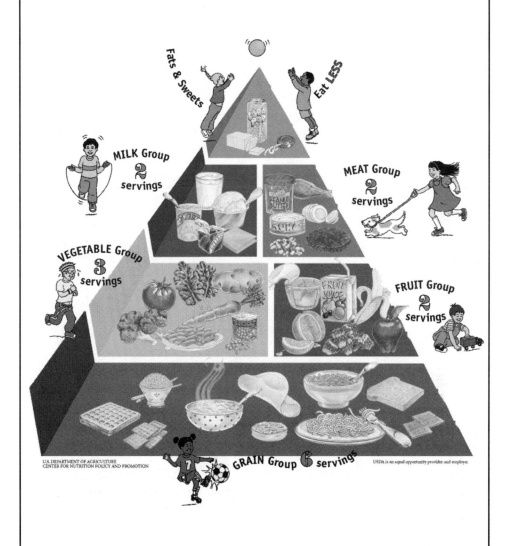

U.S. DEPARTMENT OF AGRICULTURE
CENTER FOR NUTRITION POLICY AND PROMOTION

USDA is an equal opportunity provider and employer.

Food Guide Pyramid

Ages 7 to 13
Girls Approximately 2200 calories a day
Boys Approximately 2200 calories a day

Ages 13 and up
Girls Approximately 2200 calories a day
Boys Approximately 2800 calories a day (look below for this
  symbol $\triangle$. It indicates extra servings for boys)

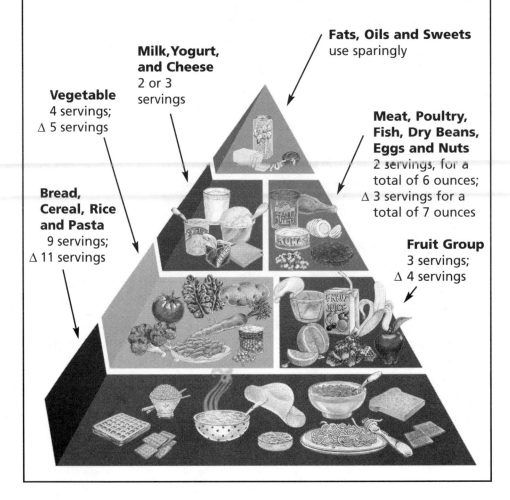

Fats, Oils and Sweets
use sparingly

**Milk, Yogurt,
and Cheese**
2 or 3
servings

Vegetable
4 servings;
$\triangle$ 5 servings

**Meat, Poultry,
Fish, Dry Beans,
Eggs and Nuts**
2 servings, for a
total of 6 ounces;
$\triangle$ 3 servings for a
total of 7 ounces

**Bread,
Cereal, Rice
and Pasta**
9 servings;
$\triangle$ 11 servings

Fruit Group
3 servings;
$\triangle$ 4 servings

One Serving Size Equals:

Breads, Cereals, Rice, Pasta
- ½ cup cooked cereal
- 1 oz ready-to-eat cereal (varies among brands)
- ½ cup cooked pasta or rice
- 1 slice of bread
- ½ English muffin
- ¼ of a 4 oz bagel

Vegetables
- 1 cup raw, leafy vegetable
- ½ cup chopped raw or cooked vegetable
- ½-¾ cup vegetable juice

Fruits
- 1 medium banana, apple, orange, or melon wedge
- ½ cup canned fruit
- ¾ cup fruit juice
- ¼ cup dried fruit

Milk, Yogurt, and Cheese
- 1 cup milk, yogurt, or pudding
- 1½-2 oz natural cheese
- 1¾ cups ice cream* or frozen yogurt*
- 2 cups cottage cheese*
    (*has a higher caloric value)

Protein: Meat, Poultry, Fish, Dry Beans, Eggs and Nuts
- 2½-3 oz of cooked lean meat, poultry, or fish
- 1 egg or 2 egg whites
- 1 oz of nuts
- 2 tablespoons peanut butter=⅓ of a serving
    (1 serving of Milk, Yogurt, or Cheese may also be used as 1 Protein serving.)

Fats, Oils, and Sweets

Limit your child's intake of calories from foods that are very high in fats, oils, or sweets (in this category, child-popular foods include: most fast foods, French fries, potato chips, fried chicken, soda, ice cream, and candy...Sorry kids!)

Most kids get sufficient quantities of fats, oils, and sugars in other foods they eat. If your child is eating too many high fat and sweet foods, it's likely he or she is skipping servings of foods from other food groups...and the foods skipped are likely the ones highest in the nutrients needed for a healthy growing body.

A child eating too many foods in this group is also at risk for childhood obesity.

 **We know children don't always eat everything you put in front of them. So an age appropriate daily multi-vitamin, just to fill in any gaps, serves as good insurance.**

Tip

What's In It For The Athlete?

The foods in each food group in the Food Guide Pyramid contain nutrients critical to the growth and healthy maturity of an active child. We all know that nutrients like Carbohydrates, Protein, and Vitamin D are important to an active child. But why, specifically?

What follows, in user-friendly bites, are the answers to these questions. Share this info with your kids. (OK. We know and you know that your goal here is to promote life-long, healthful eating habits. But all your kids need to know is that you found this really cool information about how they can score more goals at next week's soccer game. Hey, it's all in how you frame it!)

For your convenience, we've included examples of foods that are rich in each nutrient, and after each explanation you'll find all *Recommended Daily Allowances for children age 4 and up.

> **No parent or child will do this perfectly! Our lives are just too busy and our children do have their food preferences, don't they! Keep in mind, we're using words like "recommended" and "guidelines" for good reason.**
>
> **Tip**

Nutrients To Go!

Carbohydrates

Sources Include: Potatoes, Sweet Potatoes, Yams, Au Gratin Potatoes, Bread (Whole Grain Bread, Rye Bread), Cereal (Toasted Oatmeal Squares, Crispy Wheat 'N Raisins, Kix, Total, Granola, Cream of Wheat, Malt-o-Meal, Grits), Cornmeal, Rice, Wild Rice, Spanish Rice, Pasta (Spaghetti, Noodles), Chow Mein Noodles, Tortillas

Carbohydrates are the main energy source for the body. Carbohydrates are stored in the muscles and in the liver as glycogen, and in the blood as glucose (blood sugar). The body can store only limited amounts (referred to as baseline muscle storage). If an athletic activity lasts longer than two hours, and the movement is non-stop, the stored glycogen in the working muscles is depleted. If the muscles "run out of gas" (run out of glycogen) the athlete will "hit the wall and crash"; experience fatigue, weakness, light-headedness, poor concentration, and lack of coordination. Even if the athlete is not completely depleted, just low on these energy stores, injury susceptibility and performance can be affected. That's why it is so very important to nourish the body with carbohydrates before, during and after a workout or game.

On any given day, about 55-60% of a child's calories should come from carbohydrates. But on game day, we recommend increasing your child's carbohydrate intake, for all the reasons stated above. See Chapter Three, pages 47-50 for our Game Day Carbohydrate recommendations.

Protein

Sources Include: Lean meat (97% lean), Beef Jerky, Lean Pork, Poultry (skinless), Lean Turkey Burger, Pork, Fish (Halibut, Salmon, Snapper), Crab, Lobster, Peanut Butter, Mixed Nuts and Seeds, Sesame Seeds, Tofu, Lentils, Beans

Protein plays a major role in building, maintaining and repairing cells and tissues, and producing enzymes for the body. The body does not like to use protein as a main energy source, but it will if other energy reserves (carbohydrates) are low. Protein is necessary for athletes, but not in amounts above and beyond what the body needs for general good nutrition.

Note... If an athlete's carbohydrate/caloric intake is too low, and the body has no choice but to get its energy from protein (the energy needed for muscle repair and maintenance), then a child will be more susceptible to injury. And when protein stores are depleted for energy use on a regular basis, an athlete's muscle mass will decrease. Subsequently, the athlete will see a decrease in performance.

The American Dietetic Association and the USDA suggest that 12-15% of a child's calories should come from protein and that's ideal for any athletic growing child. (Follow serving recommendations on page 27.)

Fat

Sources Include: Sour Cream, Mayonnaise, Miracle Whip, Butter, Margarine, Salad Dressing (Ranch, Creamy Italian, Caesar, Blue Cheese), Vegetable Oil, Olive Oil, Canola Oil, Safflower Oil, Peanut Oil, Lard, Shortening, Flavored Crisco

Fat is a concentrated energy source that the body will use when an activity lasts longer than 20 or 30 minutes. Fat burning is critical for endurance sports. If the body's fat burning process is not working efficiently, then the body will likely use up its carbohydrate stores more quickly than is ideal, increasing the chances that the athlete will experience fatigue before the end of the event. Fat plays an essential part in some major bodily functions. For example, fat provides protection against the cold. For the kidneys and other organs, it aids in metabolizing fat-soluble vitamins A, D, E & K. Healthy fats like Omega 3 and Omega 6 fatty acids are critical for the body's manufacturing process of cell membranes, for tissue growth and blood clotting.

The American Dietetic Association and the USDA suggest 30% of a child's daily calories should come from fat. That said, on game day, watch the amount of fat in the food your child eats just prior to the start of an event, because fat takes longer to digest and too much can lead to sluggishness and an upset stomach.

Note... As a general rule of thumb, with children and adolescents, percentage of body fat should not be used as a criterion for sports participation. But, if an athlete is competing at an elite level, in a sport where ideal body fat is critical to performance, a coach or trainer may recommend that the amount of fat the child eats daily go down below 30%. If that's the advice given, we highly recommend that parents consult with a qualified health professional or nutrition expert before making any such changes in a young athlete's diet.

B$_6$ (also known as Pyridoxine)

Sources Include: Chicken, Fish, Pork, Lean Meats, Liver, Milk, Eggs, Brown Rice, Soybeans, Peanuts, Oats, Whole Wheat, Whole Grain Cereals, Nuts, Sweet Potatoes, Mixed Vegetables (Broccoli, Cabbage, Carrots), Veggie Burgers, Avocados, Bananas, Yogurt Covered Raisins, Hummus

B$_6$ is essential for the protein synthesis that occurs during rapid growth (B$_6$ level is often low in girls). It also plays a critical role in the formation of red blood cells and the healthy functioning of the brain. Typically, if the athlete eats the recommended daily amount of protein, she will also get enough B$_6$.

Recommended Daily Allowance for young children and adolescents is 1.1 mg-2.0 mg (milligrams)

B$_2$ (also known as Riboflavin)

Sources Include: Dairy Products, Beef, Poultry, Fish (Salmon, Trout, Sardines), Grains, Enriched and Fortified Cereal (Oatmeal, Apple Jacks, Apple Cinnamon and Honey Nut Cheerios), Pancakes, Waffles, Cheese, Milk, Yogurt and Frozen Yogurt, Ice Cream, Peaches, Pears, Raisins, Figs, Blueberries

An active person needs more B$_2$ than a non-active person because B$_2$ helps the body release energy from the foods we have eaten and B$_2$ is easily lost through sweat. Too much or too little B$_2$ is not recommended. This nutrient is abundant in all of the food groups. So, if a child athlete consumes a well balanced diet with the recommended servings from all food groups, a child will get plenty of B2.

Recommended Daily Allowance for young children and adolescents is 1.1 mg-1.8 mg (milligrams)

Folate (Folic Acid)

Sources Include: Green Leafy Vegetables, Legumes, Peanuts, Sunflower Seeds, Whole Grains, Bagels, Crackers, Pancakes, Waffles, Granola Bars, Oranges, Sunny Delight, Lemonade, Milk, Cheese, Liver (When was the last time your child ate liver?)

Folate helps produce red blood cells in the bone marrow, and is involved in the breakdown as well as the synthesis of proteins. A child's need for folate is increased by rapid rates of growth. If your active child does not get enough of this nutrient, the growth and repair of all cells and tissues in the body are limited. Consequences could be anemia, and/or poor growth.

Recommended Daily Allowance for young children and adolescents is 75-200 mcg (micrograms)

B₁₂ (Cobalamin)

Sources Include: Lean Ground Beef, Patty Melt, Lean Sirloin Steak, Lean Lunch Meat, Lamb Chops, Lean Ham, Pork Chops, Chicken Breast, Roasted Turkey, Dairy Products, Eggs, Egg Beaters, Liver, Fish (Tuna, Halibut, Salmon, Shrimp, Flounder), Fish Sticks, Fortified Cereals (Kix, Corn Chex, Corn Bran, Kellog's Raisin Bran, Wheaties), Many Fortified

Vegetarian Items, Tempeh, Miso, Soy Burgers, Carob Chips

A child needs plenty of B12 on hand when he or she is growing at rapid rates of speed (growth spurts). B12 helps form red blood cells in the bone marrow. B12 also plays an important role in building and maintaining the sheath that protects our nerve fibers. It helps metabolize fat, carbohydrates, and protein. B12 is essential. If there's a shortage of B12 your young athlete may be more susceptible to colds. The last thing any child wants to do is sneeze and cough while rounding second base.

*Recommended Daily Allowance for young children and adolescents is 1.0-2.0 mcg (micrograms)

Vitamin A

Sources Include: Lean Beef, Pork, Chicken, Eggs, Salmon, Shrimp, Tuna, Bass, Crab, Lobster, Milk, Custard, Ice Milk, Cheese, Asparagus, Broccoli, Swiss Chard, Kale, Spinach, Romaine Lettuce, Winter Squash, Sweet Potatoes, Pumpkins, Beans, Beets, Brussels Sprouts, Cabbage, Carrots, Celery, Lettuce, Banana Bread, Bagels, Cereals (Bran Buds, Cinnamon Toast Crunch, Golden Grahams), Apples, Apricots, Blackberries, Blueberries, Boysenberries, Cantaloupe, Cherries, Grapes, Oranges, Peaches, Pears, Plums

Vitamin A is essential for good eyesight. So this vitamin is important if your young athlete is going to see the activity around him, especially if he's playing outside at night. Vitamin A is also very important for normal body growth and formation of bone and soft tissue. Strong bones lead to a healthier athlete and to less chance of injury. Last, but certainly not least, Vitamin A helps fight infections and diseases. Less sickness means more time on the ball field.

Vitamin C

Sources Include: Lean Beef, Lamb, Pork, Poultry, Fortified Milk, Cold Cereals (100% Bran, Honey Nut Cheerios, Clusters, Cracklin' Oat Bran, Wheaties, Wheat Chex), Broccoli, Cauliflower, Green Peppers, Oranges, Apples, Bananas, Grapefruit, Peaches, Pineapple, Strawberries, Fruit Juices

Vitamin C promotes the healing of bruises, wounds, and bone fractures, all of which may be unavoidable in the life of an athlete. Vitamin C also plays a role in the formation and maintenance of collagen, a fibrous protein found in connective issues, tendons, and bones. Without it, our joints wouldn't move.

Recommended Daily Allowance for young children and adolescents is 45-60 milligrams

Vitamin E

Sources Include: Lean Poultry, Fish, Eggs, Soy Milk, Soy Beans, Tomatoes, Sweet Potatoes, Carrots, Cabbage, Asparagus, Mayonnaise, Salad Dressings, Margarine, Butter, Canola Oil, Olive Oil, Safflower Oil, Sunflower Oil, Peanuts, Sunflower Seeds, Almonds, Cashews, Hazelnuts, Pecans, Walnuts

When your daughter slides into home plate, the Vitamin E in her body will help her scraped knees heal. In addition to its role in the development of new tissue, Vitamin E acts as an antioxidant and prevents cell-membrane damage.

Recommended Daily Allowance for young children and adolescents is 7-10 Alpha Tocopherol IU (International Units)

Sodium

Sources Include: Processed Lean Meats, Milk and Dairy Products, Processed Foods, Grains, Cereals, Pickles

Sodium is the major mineral used in the regulation of fluid balance in the body.

Sodium is also needed for muscle action and nerve impulses. Sodium is very easy to get in the diet. In fact, it's much easier to get too much sodium than too little. If your child eats a healthy amount of grains, fruits, vegetables, dairy, and meat, he'll get all the sodium he needs.

Recommended Daily Allowance for young children and adolescents 300-500 mg (milligrams)

Potassium

Sources Include: Lean Beef, Lamb, Pork, Poultry, Fish, Milk, Cheese, Beans, Beets, Broccoli, Brussels Sprouts, Cabbage Carrots, Cauliflower, Celery, Corn, Mushrooms, Lettuce, Peas, Peppers, Potatoes, Soy Products, Cereals (Fiber One, Mueslix Five Grain Muesli, Raisin Bran, Grits), Cornmeal, Rice, Wheat Flour, Almonds, Chestnuts, Coconut, Hazelnuts, Peanuts, Pecans, Sesame Seeds, Sunflower Seeds, Apples, Apricots, Avocado, Bananas, Grapes, Grapefruit, Kiwi, Oranges, Peaches, Pears, Pineapple, Plums

Potassium affects fluid balance, too. It's essential for muscle function and protein synthesis. A young athlete needs adequate potassium to avoid muscle cramping.

Recommended Daily Allowance for young children and adolescents is 1400 – 2000 mg (milligrams)

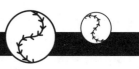

Vitamin D

Sources Include: Fortified Dairy Products, Fortified Orange Juice, Beef, Lamb, Egg Yolks, Butter, Fortified Margarine, Some Fatty Fish (Tuna, Salmon, Flounder, Snapper, Cod, Haddock, Halibut), Fortified Breads, Fortified Grains and Cereal Products, Brownies with Nuts, Sponge Cake, Apple Cobbler and Sunlight, too

Vitamin D plays a major role in the metabolism of calcium necessary for normal bone growth and development.

Recommended Daily Allowance is 10 mcg (micrograms). Put another way, for Ages 2-6, the USDA recommends a minimum of 2 servings per day of Vitamin D rich foods, for Ages 6 and up, 4 servings to meet nutritional needs. (See recommended serving sizes on page 27.)

Calcium

Sources Include: Milk, Yogurt, Cheese, Ice Cream, Fortified Cereals and Juices, Tofu, Canned Sardines, Green Leafy Vegetables, Legumes, Dried Beans and Peas, Lime-Processed Corn Tortillas, Bread, Angel Food Cake, Vanilla Wafers, Triscuits, English Muffins, Pancakes, Apples, Apricots, Cherries, Grapes, Kiwi, Bananas

Calcium is also a key player in bone development. High intake of calcium during growth and physical activity can

maximize bone mineralization. When it comes to injury susceptibility during play, we know that low calcium intake plus
repetitive force can lead to stress fractures. Calcium will also
assist in future years as a protection against osteoporosis.

Note...Adolescent athletes (and non-athletes) are at risk for
lowered calcium levels because as our kids get older we stop
pushing the milk. So, as your son or daughter enters the
teen years, be sure to encourage adequate calcium intake.

**Recommended Daily Allowance for young children and
adolescents is 800-1200 mg (milligrams)*

Fiber

*Sources Include: Fresh Fruit, Vegetables (Artichoke Hearts,
Asparagus, Corn, Yams, Radishes), All Dried Beans
(Garbanzo Beans, Black Beans, Soy Beans, etc...), Miso,
Whole Grains, Wheat Bran, Oat Bran, Banana Chips,
Oriental Snack Mix, Chocolate Coated Almonds and Peanuts*

Fiber speeds the passage of food through the digestive
track. It reduces calorie absorption and, most importantly,
may reduce exposure to cancer causing agents in the food.
Fiber also pulls fluids from the intestines as it moves
through the body. To avoid constipation, WATER, WATER,
WATER— avoiding constipation is just one of many important reasons to keep your child well hydrated.

*To Calculate Your Child's Recommended Daily Fiber Needs:
Starting with Age 2...Take child's age and add five grams of
fiber per day...So, if your child is Age 2, add 2 plus 5 grams
of fiber per day for a total of 7 grams of fiber recommended per day. If your child is 12 years old, 12 plus 5 grams of
fiber per day makes a 12 year old's total recommended
daily amount 17 grams of fiber per day.*

> **Tip**
>
> **Fiber Recommendations For Mom and Dad:** The National Cancer Institute recommends adults ingest 25 to 30 grams of fiber per day but it estimates that the average adult consumes only 11 to 23 grams per day. So eat more fiber and don't forget the water! To move everything along, 64 oz of water per day is recommended.

Iron

Sources Include: Lean Meats, Organ Meats (Liver, Kidney and Heart), Fish, Poultry, Cheese, Milk, Frozen Yogurt, Green Leafy Vegetables, Legumes, Whole Grains, Bagels, English Muffins, Granola Bars, Pretzels, Chex Mix, Trail Mix, Fruit Leather, Bread Pudding with Raisins, Peaches, Pears, Frozen Strawberries in Light Syrup, Dehydrated Pineapple

The major role of iron in the body is to make hemoglobin & myoglobin. Hemoglobin transports oxygen in our blood from the lungs to the tissues. Myoglobin transports oxygen to the muscles. Eating the recommended daily amounts of meat servings and leafy green vegetables should give a child athlete the iron she requires. If a child is a vegetarian, she should avoid eating high fiber foods at the same time she eats foods rich in iron. Fiber inhibits the absorption of iron. If she combines Vitamin C rich foods with iron rich foods, her iron absorption will be enhanced.

Note...In general, health conscious/weight conscious teens, especially girls, are at increased risk for iron deficiencies because they tend to cut out or reduce meat and dairy products from their diet.

Recommended Daily Allowance for young children and adolescents is 10 mg-12 mg (milligrams)

Zinc

Sources Include: Meat, Poultry, Pork, Lamb, Eggs, Fish, Shellfish, Chili w/Beans, Whole Wheat Saltine Crackers, Wheat Germ, Raisin Cinnamon English Muffin, Corn Nuts, Chex Mix, Milk, Frozen Yogurt, Cheddar Cheese, Swiss Cheese, American Cheese (Low Fat)

Zinc aids with functions of the immune system and plays a necessary role in enzyme production as the body metabolizes proteins, carbohydrates and fats.

It helps wounds heal, and it enhances our ability to taste our food. Children have very high zinc needs because they are growing so fast. The amount of zinc needed increases during adolescent growth spurts.

Recommended Daily Allowance of Zinc for children Age 1 to 10 is 10mg. For boys Ages 11 and up it's 15 mg (milligram) a day, for girls it's 12mg (milligrams) daily

Magnesium

Sources Include: Nuts, Seeds, Legumes, Whole Grains (not processed), Dark Green Vegetables, Bananas, Chocolate (yes, chocolate), Seafood, Pancakes, Waffles, Butter Crackers, Melba Toast, Aunt Jemima Blueberry, Buttermilk, Raisin and Whole Grain Waffles, Blueberry Pancakes

Magnesium is used by the body to promote calcium absorption, and helps in the day-to-day operation of nerves and muscles, including the heart.

Recommended Daily Allowance for young children and adolescents is 120 mg-400 mg (milligrams)

Chromium

Sources Include: Apples, Applesauce, Cantaloupe, Papaya, Broccoli, Lettuce, Mushrooms, Onions, Whole Grain Cereals, Meats

Chromium aids the protein hormone insulin in the transportation of glucose into our cells, and is involved in the cellular uptake of amino acids. Chromium aids in regulation of blood sugars. The more consistent our blood sugar level, the more consistent our energy! Energy and consistency are goals of all athletes who want to improve performance.

Recommended Daily Allowance for young children and adolescents is 50-200 mcg (micrograms)

It's Worth Repeating... Tip

If your child eats a well balanced diet, he or she will get all Recommended Daily Allowances of each nutrient.

SOURCES
* *Recommended Daily Allowances,* 10th Revised Edition, National Academy of Sciences, National Academy Press, Washington DC
* *Food Finder; Vitamin & Mineral Source Guide,* Fourth Edition, ESHA Research, Salem, OR , 1995

Chapter Three

Pre-Game Meals And Snacks

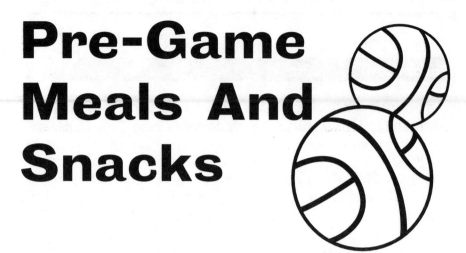

This Is The Icing On The Cake

A consistently well balanced diet is what's needed most to keep a growing, active child healthy. Subsequently, think of the Pre-Game Meal or Snack as the icing on the cake. An effective Pre-Game meal or snack can increase concentration, reduce injury susceptibility, and optimize performance.

Go Carbs, Go!

A Pre-Game meal or snack should be high in carbohydrates. Carbohydrates elevate the blood sugars needed to provide energy to all working muscles. We want energy levels up and consistent throughout a sporting event. When energy levels are constant, an athlete avoids fatigue. The less the fatigue, the better the concentration. The better the concentration, the fewer the errors on the athletic field.

Managing Game Day Jitters

Another goal of a high carb, lower fat and protein Pre-Game meal or snack is to decrease the chance of an upset stomach mid-game, all too common an occurrence when you mix food, excitement, activity, and nerves on game day. Adequate amounts of the right foods in the stomach can counter any acid buildup that may result from game day jitters.

Game Day Feeding Tips

- Your child's meal or snack eaten closest to game time should be the lightest meal of the day
- Avoid high sugar foods. They cause a sharp rise in blood sugar; a rush in energy. What goes up quickly, comes down just as fast and the child's energy level will "crash" mid-game
- Avoid trying new foods and high fiber foods on the day of a competition, especially if your child is not used to them (i.e., beans, dried fruit, etc...). Some new foods may cause stomach or intestinal problems. Try experimenting on the day of a practice instead
- Favorite or "lucky" foods are acceptable in moderation, as long as they do not cause stomach upset or create that sharp rise and fall in blood sugar
- Always allow adequate time for food to digest (follow Pre-Game Meal and Snack guidelines outlined on the next few pages)
- Keep the fat and protein to a minimum (it takes the body longer to digest fat and protein, which may increase sluggishness and the chance of an upset stomach during the game)
- If your child tends to have a "nervous stomach" on game day, consider serving a liquid meal: a "Smoothie". Smoothies digest faster, decreasing the chance of an upset stomach...and they satisfy hunger without leaving the child feeling too full. (See Chapter Seven, "Centerfield Smoothies", pages 80-93)
- Avoid carbonated beverages and caffeine. Many sodas contain caffeine, which works as a diuretic, causing the body to lose water, increasing the chances of dehydration.

Also, some nutrition experts believe carbonated beverages may induce muscle cramps

- Plan ahead so you'll have healthy foods on hand the day of a game or event. Ideally, planning ahead should minimize those last minute, high fat, fast food drive-through experiences

- When applying any nutritional advice, keep in mind that each child's individual tolerance may be different. Some children can digest a lean turkey sandwich with mustard right before a game without experiencing stomach upset or a sluggish feeling during the event. Other children, if fed within an hour of kick-off, will fare better with a sports drink and/or a plain bagel

Game Day Adjustments to Carbohydrates, Protein and Fat

Now it's time to up the Carbs! On game day you'll want to increase your child's carbohydrate intake to ensure that there's enough fuel available for all working muscles-- from kick-off through to the final play of the day. As you get closer and closer to game time, you're also going to progressively reduce fats and proteins. As you read earlier, fats and proteins take the longest to digest, and that slows everything down. So, if you don't make these adjustments before the game, you're risking sluggishness, lack of concentration, that heavy stomach feeling, and even stomach upset during play.

Please Note... All of the recommendations coming up are merely guidelines. They're based on current schools of thought in the field of Sports Nutrition, rather than on any extensive scientific study. We're simply reporting what we've seen when we've put these practices into play.

Also, you may have heard the term "Carb Loading". That's where an athlete in an endurance sport, like marathon running, starts eating carbs days before an event. That's necessary only with serious competitors and endurance athletes. (If your child is in training in an endurance sport, we recommend you seek guidance from a Sports Nutritionist before making any dietary changes beyond what we're suggesting in this chapter.)

That said... if your child has a game or strenuous workout coming up in the morning, a hearty high carbohydrate dinner and bedtime snack the night before wouldn't hurt. Then on the day of the event, just follow our high carb meal and snack guidelines, as outlined on the next few pages.

How Do You Determine Which Foods Are Good Pre-Game and Post-Game Picks?

Here's a system we've devised. Choose one of the following two methods:

1. QUICK PLAY METHOD

For Parents who do not have the time (or inclination) to calculate Grams and Carb/Protein/Fat percentages... just follow our QUICK PLAY servings recommendations, stick close to the caloric range and skip the more detailed OVERTIME METHOD completely. (See serving sizes on page 27.)

2. OVERTIME METHOD

For Parents who'd rather do the calculations themselves, use our OVERTIME METHOD as a reference guide. Then use the FDA Food Label (found on all food packages) as a point of comparison. You'll find the Calories to Grams Conversion Formula on page 171 in our Additional Resources section. Your goal is to design a Carb/Protein/Fat percentage breakdown that falls within our recommended range. You may determine if your food picks fall into our approximate range by calculating either number of grams or number of calories.

Food Label

Note... From this point on in the book, we've listed Fats/Carbs/Protein in this new order, because that's the order in which you'll find them on a Food Label.

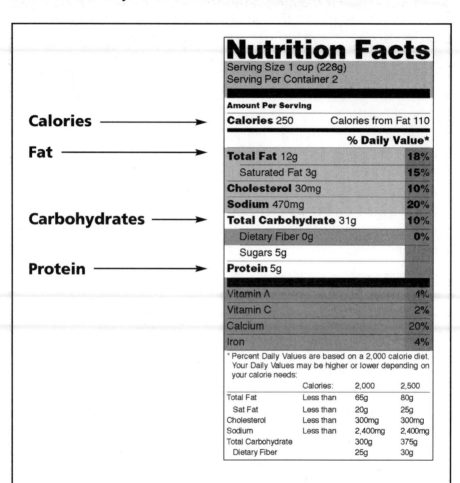

Calories ──────────→

Fat ──────────→

Carbohydrates ──────→

Protein ──────────→

Nutrition Facts

Serving Size 1 cup (228g)
Serving Per Container 2

Amount Per Serving

Calories 250   Calories from Fat 110

% Daily Value*

Total Fat 12g	**18%**
Saturated Fat 3g	**15%**
Cholesterol 30mg	**10%**
Sodium 470mg	**20%**
Total Carbohydrate 31g	**10%**
Dietary Fiber 0g	**0%**
Sugars 5g	
Protein 5g	

Vitamin A	4%
Vitamin C	2%
Calcium	20%
Iron	4%

* Percent Daily Values are based on a 2,000 calorie diet. Your Daily Values may be higher or lower depending on your calorie needs:

	Calories:	2,000	2,500
Total Fat	Less than	65g	80g
Sat Fat	Less than	20g	25g
Cholesterol	Less than	300mg	300mg
Sodium	Less than	2,400mg	2,400mg
Total Carbohydrate		300g	375g
Dietary Fiber		25g	30g

Food Label
Source: U.S. Food and Drug Administration
For more detailed instructions on how to read a Food Label, click on <u>Food Labeling and Nutrition</u> on the FDA's website, http://vm.cfsan.fda.gov

3-4 Hours Before Kick-Off
Calorie Range 700-800 calories

QUICK PLAY

Servings
1-1½ Proteins
4-5 Breads/Grains
2-3 Vegetables
0-1 Dairy
2-3 Fruits
1-2½ Fats
8-16 oz Water

Sample Meal
3 oz Roasted Chicken Breast (Boneless)
1 Whole Wheat Roll and 1½ cups Rice
1 cup Cooked Broccoli
1 Jell-O Pudding Snack (Fat Free) w/
1¼ cup of Banana Slices
1 pat of Butter
8-16 oz Water

Total
Fats 15-30%   Carbs 60-65%   Protein 12-20%

OVERTIME METHOD

Using grams or calories, combine values of all foods included in the Meal. Use Conversion Formula on page 171 to calculate ideal percentages.

	FATS	**CARBS**	**PRO**
# of Grams	12g–27g	105g–130g	21g–40g
Calorie Range	108–243 cal	420–520 cal	84–160 cal

Total
Fats 15-30%   Carbs 60-65%   Pro 12-20%

If your child eats a big meal 3 to 4 hours Pre-Game, within 30 to 90 minutes of the game, provide a 50-300 calorie snack. This will keep your child's blood sugar level as constant as possible and his or her working muscles will then have all the energy that muscles need for optimum performance. This extra calorie boost right before a game is especially important for endurance when an event is likely to last an hour or longer.

2-3 Hours Before the Game

Calorie Range 400-600 calories

QUICK PLAY

Servings	Sample Meal
½-1½ Proteins	2 oz very Lean Ground Beef
0-4 Breads/Grains	1-1½ cups Spaghetti
0-2½ Vegetables	½ cup Marinara Sauce
	¾ cup Green Beans
0-1 Dairy	½ cup Fat Free Frozen Yogurt
1-3 Fruits	1 cup Sliced Strawberries
0-2 Fats	(There's fat in meat and sauce)
8-16 oz Water	8-16 oz Water

Total

Fats 15-25%   Carbs 60-70%   Pro 12-20%

OVERTIME METHOD

Using grams or calories, combine values of all foods included in the Meal. Use Conversion Formula on page 171 to calculate ideal percentages.

	FATS	CARBS	PRO
# of Grams	7g–17g	60g–105g	12g–30g
Calorie Range	63-153 cal	240–420 cal	48–120 cal

Total

Fats 15-25%   Carbs 60-70%   Pro 12-20%

If your child eats a meal 2 to 3 hours Pre-Game, provide a 50-200 calorie snack 30 to 60 minutes before the game.

1-2 Hours Before the Game
Calorie Range 200-300 cal

QUICK PLAY

Servings
0-⅓ Proteins
0-4 Breads/Grains
0-3 Vegetables
0-2 Fruits
0-1 Fats
8-16 oz Water

Sample Meal
1 oz Fat Free Turkey Breast
2 Slices Whole Wheat Bread
(No vegetable chosen here)
20 Green Seedless Grapes
(There's a little fat in the bread)
8-16 oz Water

Total
Fats 5-15%   Carbs 65-75%   Pro 5-18%

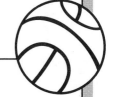

OVERTIME METHOD

Using grams or calories, combine values of all foods included in the Meal. Use Conversion Formula on page 171 to calculate ideal percentages.

	FATS	**CARBS**	**PRO**
# of Grams	1g–5g	33g–56g	3g–14g
Calorie Range	9-45 cal	132–224 cal	12–56 cal

Total
Fats 5-15%   Carbs 65-75%   Pro 5-18%

If your child is hungry right before the game, offer a piece of fruit or a sports drink.

QUICK PLAY

Servings	Sample Snack
0-½ Protein	(There's protein in the Bagel)
0-2 Grains	2 oz Whole Wheat Bagel
0-3 Vegetables	(No Vegetable chosen here)
0-½ Dairy	(No Dairy chosen here)
1-2 Fruits	½ Banana
0-½ Fat	(There's a little fat in the Bagel)
8-12 oz Water	8-12 oz Water

or

0-½ Protein	(There's protein in the Pretzel)
2 Grains	2 oz Soft Pretzel
⅓-½ serving sports drink	8 fl oz Gatorade
0-½ Fat	(There's a little fat in the Pretzel)
8-12 oz Water	8-12 oz Water

Total
Fats 0-15%   Carbs 70-100%   Pro 0-15%

OVERTIME METHOD

Using grams or calories, combine values of all foods included in the Snack. Use Conversion Formula on page 171 to calculate ideal percentages.

	FATS	CARBS	PRO
# of Grams	0g–3g	9g–50g	0g–8g
Calorie Range	0-27 cal	36–200 cal	0–32 cal

Total
Fats 0-15%   Carbs 70-100%   Pro 0-15%

Please Don't Sweat the Details!

As you are making choices based on our recommendations, it's important to understand that there is more than one way to get to the finish line. As stated earlier, the serving suggestions (food groups and serving sizes) are just guidelines. As you have seen on the last four pages, to achieve the recommended calorie ranges, and fat, carb, and protein percentages, you do not necessarily have to pick foods from every single food group listed. For example, your child may get her protein from a dairy and vegetable source (like milk and broccoli), rather than from an obvious protein source like 3 oz of chicken. Small amounts of fat may come from slices of bread or from frozen yogurt, rather than from salad dressing. Our advice is this. Using the tools we give you, try to get as close to our calorie and percentage ranges as you reasonably can. (That's what we have done with our snack suggestions in Chapters Seven through Eleven). Then give yourself some credit for trying to make sense of all of this. One of our authors, Dawn Weatherwax, studied this science for five years and has been in the field even longer... and even she thinks this stuff is complicated!

Final Assists

• These suggestions cover game day, no matter what time of day the game is scheduled to begin (morning, noon, or night). So, if your daughter likes breakfast foods better than typical lunch or dinner foods, go with her favorite breakfast foods, even if her game starts at 5 pm. The goal of the Pre-Game meal is to get your child to eat easy to digest, satisfying, healthy, high carbohydrate foods, whatever those foods may be.

- Remember, your child should drink an average of 64 oz of water daily. So add a glass of water to every meal and snack you provide
- On game day, if you're choosing a food item, or a recipe from this book (or any book), be sure to pay close attention to the FAT content. While most of our recipes are ideal when eaten as Post-Game and as everyday snacks, some recipes may be too high in fat (at 30%) for Pre-Game use. Thirty percent fat is too much fat when consumed less than 3 hours before a game or event. We can't say this often enough… too much fat right before a game can lead to sluggishness and potentially to an upset stomach!
- If one of our meal or snack recommendations contains more food than your child can eat, cut it proportionately by ¼, ⅓, or ½, and then make up the calorie difference by adding carbohydrates. The simplest way to do that is to add a sports drink or fruit juice (20 oz of Gatorade is about 150 calories, 10 oz is 75 calories)

Going the Distance

Carbohydrate intake is especially important when a young athlete participates in an event or sport that requires endurance. For example, long distance running or cycling, cross country skiing, etc…

Guidelines For Endurance Sports

When participating in a long event or practice, a young athlete should ingest 30 to 60 grams of carbohydrates per hour. Sports beverages are a best bet if the activity lasts 60 to 90 minutes. Sports drinks address both hydration and energy needs. A 20 oz sports drink (like Gatorade) equals approximately 30 to 40 grams of carbohydrates. Ideally, if the event requires staying power, additional carb intake should begin 20-30 minutes after your child begins to play.

If An Event Lasts Longer Than 90 Minutes...

Carbohydrates in solid form are also advisable. The best time to get these foods into your child is at "half-time". Some suggestions for intake of carbs in food form include: a whole wheat bagel, crackers, fruits like bananas and oranges, but not fruit juice. It's too easy to consume large amounts of fruit juice too quickly. Since fruit juice is absorbed by the body very quickly, and usually has a high sugar content, the result may be stomach upset.

Try Energy Bars

Some kids like Energy Bars. Try to find one that has the following:

- At least 7 grams of protein per serving
- A maximum of 2 to 3 grams of fat per 100 calories (calories may be listed on the food label as kcal, or kilocalories)
- Lots of <u>complex</u> carbohydrates. No more than half the carbohydrates listed on the food label should come from simple sugars. (If total carbs = 20 grams, then 10 or fewer grams should come from sugars. See food label on bar)
- Bars sweetened with brown rice syrup or that contain maltodextrin, instead of simple sugars like sugar, corn syrup, glucose, fructose, or high fructose, are preferred. Rice syrup and maltodextrin are absorbed more slowly in the body than is sugar

Many energy bars claim to be "the best", but many do not have the nutrient combination listed above. Here are some energy bars we like and we know fit our recommendations:

- Clif Bar
- Luna Bar
- PowerBar Harvest

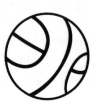

Try Sports Gels

Sports Gels, like Power Gel by PowerBar, are very, very high in carbohydrates, often 100%. Basically sports gels are carbohydrates in a "gooey" form. Many endurance athletes like these gels because they are light enough to carry on the body during events and because they absorb into the system quickly. Some people can tolerate a high percentage of carbs in this gel form, whereas the same concentration of carbs in food form would cause an upset stomach. (Again, anytime your child tries something new, plan it on the day of a practice, not on a game day…just in case.) Look for a sports gel that has maltodextrin as its main source of carbs because maltodextrin is absorbed more slowly than is glucose or fructose. Typically you'll find 25 to 30 grams of carb per sports gel which is equal to about 2 servings of breads or grains.

Post-Game Goals

Eating a high carbohydrate snack/meal after a workout is imperative!

Replenish The Energy

A high carbohydrate snack after a workout or game is essential for future optimal performance and safe play. As you read earlier, carbohydrates supply the blood sugars that are used to supply energy during a workout or game. If you don't replace the glycogen (the stored blood sugars that were just used), there won't be much in reserve for the next day's activity. This could lead to fatigue, weakness, decreased concentration, and could increase an athlete's chance of sustaining an injury. Replenishment of glycogen lost during an event is especially important if your child participates in several practices or games each week.

Timing Is Everything
The optimal time to restore glycogen (stored blood sugars) is from 30 minutes to 2 hours after intense exercise. Ideally, your child should eat a snack within thirty minutes of game's end, followed by a well balanced meal in the next 90 minutes (Fat 0-30%, Carbs 55-100%, Protein 0-25%).

Example of Ideal Timing
Practice or Game: 10:00 am to 11:30 am
Eat Carb Rich Snack: Between 11:30 am and 12 pm
Eat Carb Rich Meal: Before 1:30 pm

Ideal Post-Game Snacks
• *Official Snack Guide* Snack Recipes
• 2 pieces of fruit
• 12 oz of fruit juice (non-diluted)
• 1 oz cereal with ½ cup low fat milk, and ¼ cup raisins
• A Smoothie: 8 oz of low fat milk, crushed ice, and a medium banana. Sweeten to taste (in moderation). Blend until smooth. (Check out our Smoothie Recipes, Chapter Seven, pages 80-93.)

Why a Snack <u>and</u> a Meal?
We feed a snack right after the game because, often, kids are not very hungry right after intense exercise. It may also be a while before you can get your child to a full meal. So, an appealing snack offered within 30 minutes of game's end, followed up by a carb rich meal, is just what the coach ordered.

Note... The more intense and the longer the play, the more important it is that the child eat both a snack and a full meal within this 2 hour window.

Make Good Concession Stands

Is there a concession stand where your children play and practice? (Often, at the junior high and high school levels, team parents run a concession stand to raise extra money for the team.) If so, here's a great opportunity. Ask the people who run the stand (even if it's a professional operation), if they would consider carrying some healthy Sports Nutrition choices.

At Concession Stands:
- Thin Crust Cheese or Veggie Pizza
- Turkey Sandwiches
- Pretzels
- Baked Lay's Potato Chips
- Fresh Fruit
- Breakfast Bars
- Energy Bars
- Sports Drinks
- Lemonade
- Hot Cocoa
- 1% Milk & Skim Milk
- Refrigerated Treats (Yogurt and Pudding)
- Frozen Treats (Fudgesicles, Pudding Pops)

If the field where your children play is adjacent to a school or recreation center, and there are vending machines, you can have influence there, too. Request that these items be added to the machines:

In Soda Machines:
- Assorted Juices
- Lemonade
- Sports Drinks

In Snack Machines:
- Nuts
- Sunflower Seeds
- Healthy Trail Mix (minus candy)
- Peanut Butter & Crackers
- Cheese & Crackers
- Wheat Crackers
- Beef Jerky
- Dried Fruit
- Breakfast Bars
- Energy Bars

In Refrigerated Machines:
- Pudding
- Yogurt
- 1% Milk & Skim Milk
- Apples
- Oranges

In Ice Cream Machines:
- Fruit Juice Bars
- Pudding Pops
- Fudge Bars
- Healthy Choice Ice Cream Bars

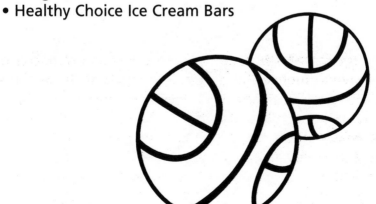

Our Position On Supplementation

Dietary supplements are not necessary for a healthy child who is eating a balanced diet! Dietary supplements will not speed up the growing process, bulk up a child's muscles, or enhance athletic performance. As a matter of fact, mega-dosing on one nutrient could affect the absorption of other nutrients needed for normal growth and energy.

A multi-vitamin (100% or less of the Recommended Daily Allowance, RDA) is the only supplementation that may be appropriate for a growing child.

If a child has a medical condition that influences what he or she can eat, diabetes for example, or if a child athlete is a vegetarian or has some other special dietary considerations, we recommend consulting with a dietitian to ensure that all nutritional needs are being met.

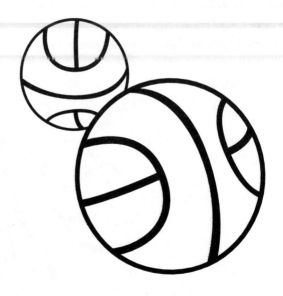

A Note About Disordered Eating And Child Athletes

Red flags should go off for parents and coaches when a child starts to cut back on eating in pursuit of some athletic goal. This is especially important to watch for if body development, body weight and body image are issues in your child's chosen sport, i.e., gymnastics, wrestling, running, swimming, dance, ice skating, cheerleading, etc.

Food restriction can lead to fatigue, dehydration, injury, and eating disorders.

At our Eating Disorders Treatment Center in Cincinnati, we're seeing an increasing number of young athletes with eating disorders. Parents and Coaches need to be especially careful about what they do and do not say to these young athletes about their body and about what they should or shouldn't eat. Even a passing comment from an influential adult about body size, shape or weight can have tremendously negative consequences if the athlete's self esteem is tied up with his or her perception of success in a given sport.

If you see or suspect that a young athlete has "disordered eating", seek professional advice. Eating disorders rarely go away without professional help.

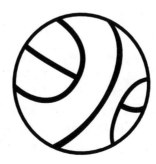

Chapter Four

10 Minutes To Kick-Off:

Grocery Store Pick-Ups On The Run

No food in the house. No time before the game. The kids are screaming in the back seat of your car. You have to feed them something before the game... and you have to have a snack on hand when the game's over. Your only option is to pick something up on-the-fly, so you find the closest supermarket or convenience store on the way to the ball field.

Note... We know you're busy. But we just wanted to say that the food suggestions in this chapter are also good snack picks, even if they're bought ahead of time, and are taken to the game in a leisurely sort of way.

Pre-Game/Post-Game Draft Picks

♥ = An example of a good high carb selection for Pre-Game, Post-Game, or both. Selections in the latter part of this list are too high in fat, sugar, or protein to be eaten right before a game or practice, but they are ideal for post-game snacking.

Once you are familiar with the types of foods we're recommending here, you'll be able to compare food labels and pick out many similar items in your supermarket.

With all foods recommended on our list, follow the package instructions for 1 serving size. (When you're not in a rush, teach your children what you're looking for and let them find the serving size and the Fat, Carb and Protein values on the food labels.)

FOOD ITEM Serving Size=1	PRE GAME Less than 1 hr. before game	POST GAME Within 30 min. of activity's end
Grapes (15-20 grapes)	♥	♥
Banana (1 medium)	♥	♥
Apple (1 medium)	♥	♥
Orange or Tangerine	♥	♥
Fresh Fruit From Salad Bar (l cup)	♥	♥
Del Monte/Dole Individual Fruit Cups (in water)	♥	♥
MOTT'S Apple Sauce (individual containers)	♥	♥
Stretch Island Fruit Leather	♥	♥
SUNSWEET Fruitlings	♥	♥
JELL-O Gelatin Snacks	♥	♥
Kraft Handi Snack Apple Dippers	♥	♥
Dole Fruit 'N Juice Bars	♥	♥
Betty Crocker Fruit Snacks (Scooby-Doo, Lucky-Charms & Hawaiian Punch)	♥	♥

FOOD ITEM Serving Size=1	PRE GAME Less than 1 hr. before game	POST GAME Within 30 min. of activity's end
Baby Carrots	♥	♥
V8 Splash (Grape Blend, Tropical Blend)	♥	♥
Baked Tostitos	♥	♥
New York Style Bagel Chips	♥	♥
Mini Bagels	♥	♥
Goldfish (pretzel flavor)	♥	♥
Manischewitz Bagel Pretzels (All varieties)	♥	♥
Keebler Snackin Grahams	♥	♥
Orville Redenbacher's Caramel Mini Rice Cakes	♥	♥
Hain Pure Foods Kidz Animal Crackers (Honey & Chocolate)	♥	♥
Hain Pure Foods Crispetts (Original, Cheese)	♥	♥
Kellogg's Crispix	♥	♥
Kraft, JELL-O, & Hunt's Fat-Free Pudding Snacks	♥	♥
Dannon Sprinkl'ins	♥	♥
Fudgesicle	♥	♥
Gatorade	♥	♥
POWERaDE	♥	♥
ALL SPORT	♥	♥
Raisin Boxes (Store Brands)		♥
SUN MAID Dried Fruits, Figs		♥

FOOD ITEM Serving Size=1	PRE GAME Less than 1 hr. before game	POST GAME Within 30 min. of activity's end
SUNSWEET (or Store Brand) Pitted Prunes		♥
Ocean Spray Craisins		♥
Dole Cinna Raisin		♥
Transverse Bay Fruit Co. Dried Fruit (Berry & Cherry, Blueberries, Cranberries)		♥
Fresh Fruit with Fruit Dip		♥
Golden Stream Trail Mix (with fruit and nuts, no candy)		♥
Country Choice Oatmeal Raisin Cookies		♥
Pre-cut Veggies with Light Ranch Dressing		♥
Baked Tostitos (various kinds) with Salsa		♥
Guiltless Gourmet Baked Tortilla Chips (Blue Corn, Spicy Black Bean, Yellow Corn)		♥
Nabisco Oyster Crackers		♥
Sunbelt Banana Nut Granola Cereal		♥
Chex-Mix (Original, Ranch, Honeynut)		♥
Orville Gourmet Low-Fat Popcorn		♥
Air Crisps (Cheese Nips, Wheat Thin, Pretzel, Potato, Original)		♥
Vanilla Wafers		♥
Nature Valley 100% Natural Granola Bars (all flavors)		♥

FOOD ITEM Serving Size=1	PRE GAME Less than 1 hr. before game	POST GAME Within 30 min. of activity's end
Power Bar		♥
Luna Bar		♥
Clif Bar		♥
Power Bar Essentials		♥
Nutri-Grain Bar		♥
String Cheese		♥
Yoplait Yumsters		♥
Yoplait Go-Gurt		♥
Minute Maid Orange or Apple Juice		♥
Everfresh Orange or Apple Juice		♥
Juicy Juice Individual Juice Box		♥
MOTT'S Individual Juice Box		♥
Hi-C Individual Juice Box (apple, cherry, orange)		♥

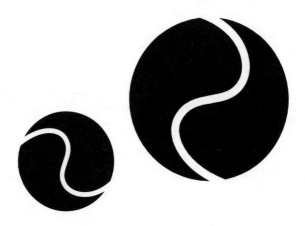

Last Minute Huddle

- Before, during, or after a game, if you ever find yourself in a situation where you cannot purchase any of the above items (all that's between you and the ball field is a 7-Eleven), remember <u>some</u> carbohydrates are better than none. Hard candy, licorice, gummy bears, Hot Tamales, or similar items, are a better choice than a high fat, high protein, candy bar or cookie. But beware...with any high sugar food your child's blood sugars could rise and fall quickly. So moderation is the key. If candy is the only option, buy some peanuts, too. Take 1 oz of peanuts and mix with 4 oz of candy. The combination will slow down the quick rise in blood sugar

- One of the simplest, most efficient ways to get carbs into a child Pre-Game is with a sports drink or a diluted fruit juice.

- As mentioned earlier, always try to pick a fruit juice that has the highest amount of Vitamin C and percentage of real fruit juice in the ingredients (remember to dilute with 2x water)

- Obviously, pre-planning is the best game plan. Once you know which Sports Nutrition snacks your children like best, you can keep them on hand in quantity, and avoid this "Pick-Ups On The Run" Chapter altogether. (If only family life could run so smoothly...)

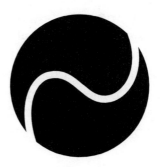

Chapter Five

Score Points In The Drive-Through Lane

When "FAST FOOD" Is All You've Got

There's no time to prepare a meal. Your child must be fed before the game. And the honest truth is this...sometimes fast food is all your child will eat and you just do not have the time or energy to fight.

Our Tips For Making The Best of Life in the "Fast Food" Lane

- If you know in advance that your schedule will necessitate a drive-through breakfast, lunch or dinner before a game, plan to balance the rest of your child's daily intake with low fat, high carbohydrate choices
- With salads, order low fat dressings, or have regular dressing put on the side. Salad dressing can add an additional 400 calories of fat to your child's meal, which may cause sluggishness immediately following the meal
- Request all special sauces, butter, sour cream and cheese on the side and encourage your child to use them sparingly
- Order grilled rather than fried foods
- Order a baked potato instead of fries

- Order regular size items rather than super size or large
- Order nonfat or 1% milk instead of whole milk
- If your teenager usually orders two sandwiches, replace one with a salad, or a low fat milk, or a low fat shake
- Some day when you are not in a hurry, go to your nearby fast food restaurants and ask for nutrition pamphlets. Read them before the next time you order. Then you can make more informed choices regarding calories, carbohydrates, protein and fat content
- If the caloric value of any of your fast food choices is too high, based on time proximity to your child's game or practice, do a little calorie cutting—cut the meal by a quarter, or a third, or a half

Let's face it. Today, it's a rare parent who can completely do away with fast food in his or her child's world. So turn the battle into an opportunity...help your child become an informed participant in this whole process. Share with him or her whatever you're learning about how to make healthier fast food choices. Ultimately, your intent here is to help your son or daughter make healthy food choices, even (especially) when you're not around.

Much of what you'll find at a fast food restaurant will be high in saturated fats, sodium and grease, and low in nutrients. Much, but not all.

Coming up on pages 69-75 are examples of some "healthier" options available at several popular fast food chains. These choices range in caloric value. Our suggestions include a variety of breakfast, lunch and dinner foods. These meals do not always fit within our Pre-Game and Post- Game guidelines. But they are the best we (and you) can do if fast food is your only option.

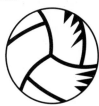

Remember Timing of Pre-Game Meals and Snacks

PREGAME `3-4 HRS`

700-800 cal   *Fats 15-30%*   *Carbs 60-65%*   *Pro 12-20%*

PREGAME `2-3 HRS`

400-600 cal   *Fats 15-25%*   *Carbs 60-70%*   *Pro 12-20%*

PREGAME `1-2 HRS`

200-300 cal   *Fats 5-15%*   *Carbs 65-75%*   *Pro 5-18%*

PREGAME `<1 HOUR`

50-200 cal   *Fats 0-15%*   *Carbs 70-100%*   *Pro 0-15%*
(Depends on individual tolerance)

POST **GAME**

Snacks 100-300 cal
Meals 400-600 cal
         Fats 0-30%   *Carb 55-100%*   *Pro 0-25%*

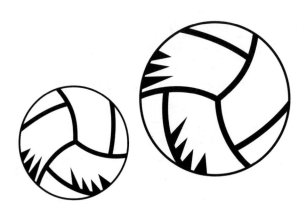

Our "On The Road" Picks

These are examples! When these choices fit closely enough to our Pre-Game Guidelines, you'll see our Pre-Game Icons with a timing suggestion. You'll see the Post-game Icon with all of our choices because all work as Post-Game Meals. (Wherever applicable, our nutrition values include standard hamburger and sandwich toppings.)

McDonald's

PREGAME 3-4 HRS **POST GAME**

Order of Hotcakes w/2 Pats Butter and Syrup, 1% Milk and 6 oz Orange Juice
Calories 803   Fat 21%   Carb 70%   Pro 9%

PREGAME 3-4 HRS **POST GAME**

Egg McMuffin (English Muffin with Jelly would be better if your child will eat it), 1% Milk and 6 oz Orange Juice
Calories 507   Fat 27%   Carb 52%   Pro 21%

PREGAME 2-3 HRS **POST GAME**

Hamburger, Garden Salad w/2 Tablespoons Fat-Free Herb Vinaigrette Dressing and Vanilla Ice Cream Cone
Calories 495   Fat 25%   Carb 60%   Pro 15%

PREGAME 3-4 HRS **POST GAME**

Grilled Chicken Deluxe, Small French Fries and Strawberry Sundae
Calories 800   Fat 24%   Carb 57%   Pro19%

Burger King

PREGAME 3-4 HRS   **POST** GAME

Hamburger, 10 oz Orange Juice and Medium Vanilla Shake
Calories 770   Fat 25%   Carb 59%   Pro 16%

Wendy's

PREGAME 2-3 HRS   **POST** GAME

Small Chili, Plain Baked Potato and Side Salad
w/1 Tablespoon Reduced Fat Salad Dressing
(Warning...This selection may be too high in fiber for
a child who is not used to a food like Chili)
Calories 610   Fat 19%   Carb 64%   Pro 17%

PREGAME 3-4 HRS   **POST** GAME

Grilled Chicken Sandwich, a Breadstick, Side Salad w/1
Tablespoon Reduced Fat Salad Dressing and Small Frosty
Calories 870   Fat 25%   Carb 56%   Pro 19%

PREGAME 3-4 HRS   **POST** GAME

Hamburger, Side Salad w/1 Tablespoon Reduced Ranch
Dressing and Small Frosty
Calories 810   Fat 33%   Carb 49%   Pro 18%

Hardee's

PREGAME 2-3 HRS **POST** GAME

2 Apple Cinnamon 'n' Raisin Biscuits and 10 oz Orange Juice
Calories 640   Fat 22%   Carb 74%   Pro 4%

PREGAME 2-3 HRS **POST** GAME

Grilled Chicken Sandwich, Mashed Potatoes
and Cool Twist Cone
Calories 606   Fat 21%   Carb 59%   Pro 20%

Whataburger

PREGAME 2-3 HRS **POST** GAME

3 Pancakes, 2% Milk and 10 oz Orange Juice
Calories 512   Fat 18%   Carb 66%   Pro 16%

PREGAME 3-4 HRS **POST** GAME

Chicken Fajita, Garden Salad w/1 Tablespoon Low Fat Ranch
Dressing and 2% Milk
Calories 507   Fat 25%   Carb 52%   Pro 23%

PREGAME 3-4 HRS **POST** GAME

Grilled Chicken w/o Bun, Garden Salad w/1 Packet
Low Fat Vinaigrette and 2% Milk
Calories 593   Fat 20%   Carb 50%   Pro 30%

PREGAME 3-4 HRS **POST** GAME

Grilled Chicken Salad w/1 Tablespoon Reduced Fat Ranch
Dressing, Texas Toast and 12 oz Chocolate Shake
Calories 734   Fat 22%   Carb 58%   Pro 20%

Dairy Queen

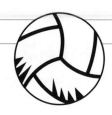

POST GAME

Banana Split
Calories 410   Fat 21%   Carb 73%   Pro 61%

Medium Chocolate Sundae
Calories 510   Fat 22%   Carb 70%   Pro 8%

DQ Fudge Bar
Calories 70   Fat 0%   Carb 76%   Pro 24%

DQ Sandwich
Calories 150   Fat 29%   Carb 63%   Pro 8%

DQ Vanilla Orange Bar
Calories 75   Fat 0%   Carb 89%   Pro 11%

Domino's

PREGAME 2-3 HRS **POST** GAME

3 Slices Thin Crust Cheese Pizza With Mushrooms, Skim Milk
and Side Salad w/3 Tablespoons Lite Italian Dressing
Calories 528   Fat 27%   Carb 56%   Pro 17%

Fazoli's

PREGAME 2-3 HRS **POST GAME**

Spaghetti w/ Meat Sauce, Garden Salad w/2 Tablespoons
Reduced Calorie Italian Dressing and Minestrone Soup
Calories 559   Fat 21%   Carb 59%   Pro 20%

PREGAME 3-4 HRS **POST GAME**

Broccoli and Fettuccine, Bean and Pasta Soup, and Lemon
Italian Ice
Calories 740   Fat 24%   Carb 64%   Pro 12%

Dunkin Doughnuts

PREGAME 1-2 HRS **POST GAME**

Any Low Fat Muffin and 1% milk
Calories ~360   Fat 11%   Carb 73%   Pro 16%

PREGAME 3-4 HRS **POST GAME**

2 Glazed Donuts and 10 oz Orange Juice
Calories 580   Fat 28%   Carb 64%   Pro 5%

PREGAME 3-4 HRS **POST GAME**

2 Blueberry Cake Donuts or 2 Blueberry Crumb Donuts
and Skim Milk
Calories 460   Fat 30%   Carb 63%   Pro 7%

Bruegger's Bagels

PREGAME 1-2 HRS | **POST GAME**

Bagel w/Light Cream Cheese and 16 oz Orange Juice
(Any Bagel except, "Cinnamon", "Everything", or "Salt")
Calories 590   Fat 11%   Carb 79%   Pro 10%

PREGAME 3-4 HRS | **POST GAME**

Chicken Fajita Bagel Sandwich and 1% Milk
Calories 580   Fat 19%   Carb 54%   Pro 27%

Carl's Jr.

PREGAME 2-3 HRS | **POST GAME**

Jr. Hamburger and Plain Baked Potato w/2 packets of Salsa
Calories 640   Fat 19%   Carb 66%   Pro 15%

Pizza Hut

PREGAME 3-4 HRS | **POST GAME**

3 Slices Large Chicken Veggie Pizza (The Edge)
Calories 480   Fat 30%   Carb 55%   Pro 15%

PREGAME 3-4 HRS | **POST GAME**

3 Slices Medium Veggie Lover's Pizza, Hand Tossed Crust
Calories 720   Fat 26%   Carb 56%   Pro 18%

Arby's

PREGAME 2-3 HRS **POST GAME**

Blueberry Muffin, Hot Chocolate and 6 oz Orange Juice
Calories 442   Fat 20%   Carb 76%   Pro 4%

PREGAME 2-3 HRS **POST GAME**

1 Roast Chicken Deluxe, Garden Salad w/4 Tablespoons
Reduced Calorie Italian Dressing and 6 oz Orange Juice
Calories 439   Fat 16%   Carb 62%   Pro 22%

Subway

PREGAME 2-3 HRS **POST GAME**

6" Roasted Chicken Breast Sub, Veggie Delite Salad w/2
Tablespoons or ½ Packet Fat-Free Ranch Dressing and Bag
Baked Lay's Chips
Calories 591   Fat 15%   Carb 65%   Pro 20%

PREGAME 2-3 HRS **POST GAME**

6" Subway Club, Veggie Delite Salad w/2 Tablespoons or ½
Packet Fat-Free Ranch Dressing and 1 Oatmeal Raisin Cookie
Calories 597   Fat 21%   Carb 62%   Pro 17%

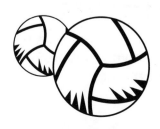

Chapter Six

How To Use Our Snack Recipes

Any Child, Any Snack, Anytime!

All of the recipes in Chapters Seven through Eleven have been tested on children. (No children were harmed during the making of this book, we promise.) Not surprisingly, we found that all kids, even those not participating in sports, liked our snacks. So, if you're looking for "all occasion" snack ideas for any child, anytime, every one of our recipes will fit the bill.

For The "Athlete" In Your House

If your young "athlete" has a practice or a game coming up in a few hours, slide into "Sports Nutrition" mode...and use the sidebars located to the left or right of each recipe.

Again, our goal here is to give you the tools you need to make good food choices for your child, Pre and Post-Game. Please use our recomendations as guiding principles, not as "absolute" rules.

In the sidebars next to each snack recipe you'll find examples of food and drink you may serve with the snack, to make each snack even more versatile, Sports Nutrition-wise.

Remember, as we get closer and closer to game time we want to progressively increase carbohydrate intake (for energy), while reducing the fat and protein (to avoid stomach distress and sluggishness). Post-Game, our primary goal is to get a high carb snack into your child, to replenish energy lost.

Look For Our Recommendations

PREGAME 3-4 HRS

700-800 cal   Fats 15-30%   Carbs 60-65%   Protein 12-20%

PREGAME 2-3 HRS

400-600 cal   Fats 15-25%   Carbs 60-70%   Protein 12-20%

PREGAME 1-2 HRS

200-300 cal   Fats 5-15%   Carbs 65-75%   Protein 5-18%

PREGAME < 1 HOUR

50-200 cal   Fats 0-15%   Carbs 70-100%   Protein 0-15%

POST GAME

Snacks 100-300 cal
Meals 400-600 cal

Fats 0-30%   Carbs 55-100%   Protein 0-25%

Information In Sports Nutrition Sidebars

Sidebar example

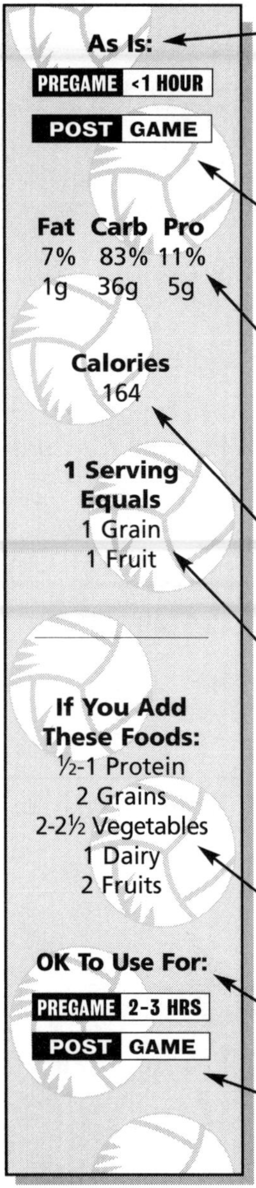
As Is:
PREGAME <1 HOUR
POST GAME
Fat Carb Pro
7% 83% 11%
1g 36g 5g
Calories
164
1 Serving
Equals
1 Grain
1 Fruit
If You Add
These Foods:
½-1 Protein
2 Grains
2-2½ Vegetables
1 Dairy
2 Fruits
OK To Use For:
PREGAME 2-3 HRS
POST GAME

- **"As Is"**, with no other foods added, this snack is a good selection for the specific Pre-Game and/or Post-Game times listed (Based on percentages of Fats, Carbs, and Protein)
- **Time icons** give specific time recommendations, Pre-Game and Post-Game
- **Fat, Carbs, and Protein** values are listed in both percentages and grams
- **Calories** per serving
- **Number of servings** from each Food Group found in **1 serving** of this snack
- **If You Add These Foods,** this snack becomes
- **OK To Use For** these specific
- **Pre or Post-Game times**

As you become more familiar with the food groups and serving sizes, as outlined in our QUICK PLAY METHOD (pages 45-50), you'll become skilled at figuring out how to make these adjustments yourself.

Note... All nutritional values are based on 1 serving size. For example, if a recipe serves 4, one-fourth of the recipe equals 1 serving. If a recipe makes 12 pieces of cake, one-twelfth equals one serving.

All percentages were rounded to the nearest number.

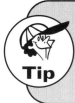

Remember, if you'd like to do your own Calories to Grams (or Grams to Calories) calculations, we've included that Conversion Formula in our Additional Resources Section, page 171.

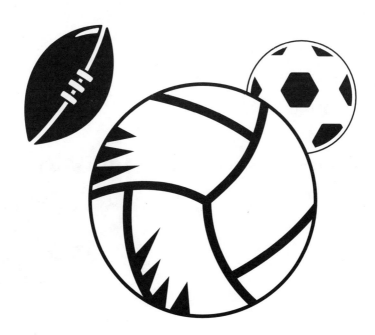

Chapter Seven

Centerfield Smoothies

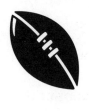

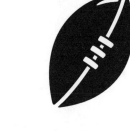

Berry Banana Blitz

Banana Honey Hat Trick

Match Point Milk Shakes & Malts

Slam Dunk Chocolate Soy Shake

Triple Play Chocolate-Almond-Marshmallow Madness

Slap Shot Banana Smoothie

Ron's Pineapple Power Pitch

Fast Break Cantaloupe Shake

First Down Fruit & Soy Frostee

Multi-Fruit Marathon

Open-Ice Orange Creamsicle

Strawberry Banana Soy Sensation

Peach Berry Bank Shot

Berry Banana Blitz

1 banana
1 container, 8 oz, low fat vanilla yogurt
1 pkg., 10 oz, frozen strawberries,
   unsweetened, thawed
¼ cup orange juice
1 tablespoon honey

Cut banana into chunks. Place into
blender with all other ingredients.
Cover and blend until smooth.

Serves 3

When adding foods for Pre-Game and Post-Game versatility, it may be helpful to refer back to our "One Serving Size Equals:" information on page 27. Tip

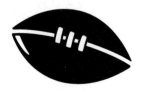

Fat	Carb	Pro
7%	83%	11%
1g	36g	5g

Calories
164

1 Serving Equals
1 Grain
1 Fruit

If You Add These Foods:
½-1 Protein
2 Grains
2-2½ Vegetables
1 Dairy
2 Fruits

OK To Use For:
PREGAME 2-3 HRS
POST GAME

Fat Carb Pro

6%   82%   10%

2g   45g   6g

Calories
200

1 Serving
Equals
½ Dairy
2 Fruits

If You Add
These Foods:
1-1¼ Grains

OK To Use For:
PREGAME **1-2 HRS**

POST **GAME**

Banana Honey Hat Trick

2 bananas
1 cup low fat soy milk
1 tablespoon honey
¾ to 1 teaspoon vanilla extract
6-8 ice cubes

Cut bananas into chunks. In blender combine bananas, milk, honey and vanilla. Cover and blend until smooth. Add ice cubes, 2 at a time. Cover and blend again until smooth.

Serves 2

Tip

Honey sometimes turns "grainy" when stored. To make it pourable again, heat honey container in microwave for several seconds.

Match Point Milk Shakes & Malts

½ cup skim milk
2 cups nonfat frozen vanilla yogurt
1 teaspoon vanilla extract

Place all ingredients in blender. Cover and blend until smooth.

Variations:
- *Old Fashioned Malt:*
  Add 1 tablespoon malt powder
- *Chocolate Shake:*
  Add 1 tablespoon chocolate syrup

Serves 2

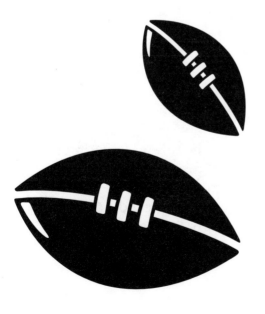

As Is:

POST GAME

Fat	Carb	Pro
2%	75%	21%
0g	41g	12g

Calories
218
vanilla;
260
w/malt powder;
290
w/chocolate

1 Serving Equals
2½ Grains
¼ Dairy

If You Add These Foods:
1 Protein
2 Grains
2 Vegetables
3 Fruits
1 Fat

OK To Use For:

PREGAME 3-4 HRS

POST GAME

As Is:

PREGAME 1-2 HRS

POST GAME

Fat Carb Pro
8%   79%   14%
2g   44g   8g

Calories
222

1 Serving Equals
2 Grains
1 Dairy

If You Add These Foods:
½ Protein
½ Grain
2-2½ Vegetables
2 Fruits

OK To Use For:

PREGAME 2-3 HRS

POST GAME

Slam Dunk Chocolate Soy Shake

⅓ cup chocolate syrup
1½ cups plain low fat soy milk
4 ice cubes

Place all ingredients and ice in blender. Cover and blend until smooth.

Serves 2

Tip

Soy milk gives a smoothie a creamy richness that you won't get when you use skim milk. In any smoothie recipe, you may substitute soy milk for skim milk, in equal measure. Soy milk comes plain and in flavors like vanilla and chocolate. Experiment. Use soy milk instead of skim milk in a smoothie that you've made before. See if your child notices any flavor change. Soy milk does have its own distinctive taste.

Triple Play Chocolate-Almond-Marshmallow Madness

Fat	Carb	Pro
3%	89%	8%
1g	65g	6g

Calories
287

1/3 cup chocolate syrup
1 cup skim milk
1/8 teaspoon almond extract
1/2 cup marshmallow creme
1/4 cup silk or silken, low fat tofu
4 ice cubes

Place chocolate syrup, milk, almond extract, marshmallow creme, and tofu in blender. Cover and blend until smooth. Add ice cubes, cover, and blend again until smooth. If preferred, it's OK to make without the almond extract.

1 Serving Equals
3 Grains
1/2 Dairy

Serves 2

If You Add These Foods:
1 Protein
2-2½ Vegetables
1 Fruit

OK To Use For:
PREGAME 2-3 HRS
POST GAME

Tip

Are you "tofu-phobic"? We understand. Tofu is a white, slippery, jiggly blob of soy that comes packed in water. While it's certainly unappealing to look at, it is a wonderful source of protein, calcium, B vitamins, iron and zinc! With virtually no flavor of its own, tofu takes on the flavor of whatever you mix with it. In addition to being incredibly healthy, tofu will make your smoothies rich and creamy! It comes in 4 consistencies. Be sure to use "silk" or "silken" tofu in all smoothie recipes. It's the softest and will blend best.

Fat Carb Pro
7%   75%   18%
2g   36g   9g

Calories
185

**1 Serving
Equals**
1 Dairy
1 Fruit

**If You Add
These Foods:**
½ Protein
2½ Grains
2 Vegetables
1 Fruit
1 Fat

OK To Use For:

PREGAME 2-3 HRS

POST GAME

Slap Shot
Banana Smoothie

2 bananas
1½ cups skim milk
1 carton, 8 oz, low fat vanilla yogurt
2 teaspoons powdered sugar
4 ice cubes

Cut bananas into chunks. In blender combine bananas, milk, yogurt and sugar. Cover and blend until smooth. Add ice cubes, cover and blend again until smooth.

Serves 3

> **Tip**
>
> For a variation on the all banana theme, occasionally pinch hit with strawberry-banana yogurt or a citrus flavor yogurt. Be as adventuresome as your child will allow.

Ron's Pineapple Power Pitch

1 banana
1 cup pineapple juice
⅓ cup nonfat instant dry powdered milk
2-3 tablespoons granulated sugar
1 teaspoon vanilla extract
8-10 ice cubes

Cut banana into chunks. Place into blender with pineapple juice, powdered milk, sugar, vanilla and 4 ice cubes. Cover and blend until smooth. Add remaining ice cubes, a few at a time and blend again, covered, until smooth.

Serves 2

Pineapple is a bone builder. It contains Manganese which helps build connective tissues, bone, skin and cartilage.

Tip

As Is:

PREGAME 1-2 HRS

POST GAME

Fat	Carb	Pro
2%	88%	8%
0g	57g	5g

Calories
247

1 Serving Equals
1 Grain
½ Dairy
2 Fruits

If You Add These Foods:
1 Protein
4 Grains
2 Vegetables
½ Dairy
1 Fat

OK To Use For:

PREGAME 3-4 HRS

POST GAME

Fat Carb Pro
7% 82% 11%
1g 37g 5g

Calories
166

**1 Serving
Equals**
1½ Grains
1 Fruit

**If You Add
These Foods:**
1 Grain
½ Fruit or
4-8 oz Sports
Drink

OK To Use For:

PREGAME 1-2 HRS

POST GAME

Fast Break Cantaloupe Shake

½ medium-sized cantaloupe
1 tablespoon fresh lemon juice
1 tablespoon honey
¾ cup low fat vanilla frozen yogurt

Scoop out and discard the cantaloupe seeds. With a spoon, scoop fruit from melon and toss into a blender or food processor. Add lemon juice, honey and frozen yogurt. Blend until mixture is smooth.

Serves 2

Be exotic! Instead of melon, use mango, papaya or other seasonal fruits. A smoothie is a great way to get your children to try new fruits.

Tip

First Down Fruit & Soy Frostee

5 oz silk or silken tofu
2 cups fresh or frozen fruit, your choice
¾ teaspoon vanilla extract
1½ tablespoons honey

Combine the above ingredients in a blender. Cover and blend until smooth.

Serves 2

Tip While storing tofu in your refrigerator, be sure the tofu is immersed in water. If you change the water daily, tofu should last for 1 week.

As Is:

PREGAME	<1 HOUR
POST	GAME

Fat Carb Pro
15% 72% 12%
2g   26g   4g

Calories
134

1 Serving Equals
½ Protein
1 Grain
1 Fruit

If You Add These Foods:
1-1¼ Grains
½-1 Fruit

OK To Use For:

PREGAME	1-2 HRS
POST	GAME

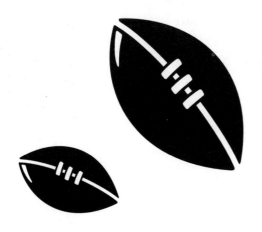

Multi-Fruit Marathon

2 tablespoons cold water
2 ripe peaches or nectarines, peeled and chopped, or
½ cup raspberries, and
¾ cup strawberries (you may use a mixture of any of the above)
⅓ cup instant nonfat dry milk powder
1 cup ice cubes

Blend water and fruit. Add the nonfat dry milk powder and ice cubes. Blend until consistency is rich and frothy.

Serves 1

Tip

Nonfat dry milk powder is an excellent source of calcium. Stored in your refrigerator or freezer it will last for months.

Open-Ice
Orange Creamsicle

1 can, 6 oz, frozen orange juice
    concentrate
1 teaspoon orange zest (optional)
8 oz low fat or nonfat plain yogurt
1 teaspoon vanilla extract
2½ cups skim or 1% milk

Mix all of the above ingredients in a
blender. Cover and blend until smooth.

(Nutrition values were calculated with
low fat yogurt.)

Serves 6

"Zest" is the finely grated colored
peel of the fruit. Orange and
lemon zest are frequently
used in recipes to add flavor.

Tip

As Is:
POST GAME

Fat	Carb	Pro
14%	64%	21%
1g	19g	6g

Calories
115

1 Serving Equals
1 Fruit
1 Dairy

If You Add These Foods:
1 Protein
3 Grains
1 Fruit
1 Fat

OK To Use For:
PREGAME 2-3 HRS

POST GAME

PREGAME <1 HOUR

POST GAME

Fat Carb Pro
12% 77% 11%
2g   26g   4g

Calories
126

**1 Serving
Equals**
3 Vegetables
1 Fruit

**If You Add
These Foods:**
2 Grains

OK To Use For:

PREGAME 1–2 HRS

POST GAME

Strawberry Banana Soy Sensation

3 cups plain or vanilla soy milk
1 banana
1 cup strawberries

Place all ingredients in blender. Cover and blend until smooth.

Serves 4

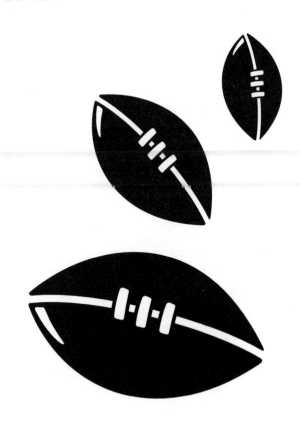

Peach Berry Bank Shot

1 pkg., 16 oz, frozen unsweetened
 sliced peaches or nectarines
⅔ cup frozen unsweetened
 whole strawberries
1½ cups skim or fat-free milk
1½ tablespoons honey
1½ cups plain fat-free yogurt
1 teaspoon vanilla extract
⅛ teaspoon cinnamon

Place all ingredients in a blender.
Cover and blend. Stop blender and
stir occasionally. Continue blending
until mixture is thick and smooth.

Serves 5

Use fresh strawberries,
or peeled peaches or nec-
tarines, when available.

Tip

Chapter Eight

Pre-Game Breakfasts To Go!

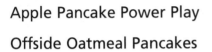

Apple Pancake Power Play

Offside Oatmeal Pancakes

All Star Apple-Raisin Breakfast Sandwich

Center Court Waffles with Dribble Toppings

Banana Wheat Germ MVP Muffins

Granola-Almond Marching Muffins

Freestyle Cinnamon Apple Oat Bran Muffins

Banana Kick Bread

M.C.'s Blueberry Break Coffee Cake

Five-Minute Free Agent Omelet

Eggs-treme Cheese Burrito

Half-Time Hot Chocolate

Apple Pancake Power Play

3 tablespoons sugar
¾ teaspoon cinnamon
¼ teaspoon nutmeg
⅛ teaspoon salt
1 cup all-purpose flour
1 tablespoon soy flour
2 teaspoons baking powder
¾ cup soy milk
1 teaspoon vanilla extract
2 tablespoons margarine or liquid
  vegetable spread
1 tart apple, peeled, cored, then
  grated or finely chopped

TOPPINGS: ¼ cup applesauce or 3
  tablespoons lite maple syrup

Blend sugar with cinnamon, nutmeg, and salt. Blend sugar mixture with all-purpose flour, soy flour, and baking powder. In a separate bowl, whisk together the soy milk, vanilla extract, and margarine. Add apples and dry mix and gently blend. Pour ¼ cup of batter onto a hot non-stick griddle or pan. Cook for 2 minutes on the first side or until bubbles appear on the surface. Flip and cook for another minute, or until heated through. Top each serving with ¼ cup applesauce or 3 tablespoons lite maple syrup.

Makes 12 pancakes;
serving size 2 pancakes

As Is:

PREGAME 1-2 HRS

POST GAME

Fat Carb Pro
18% 75% 7%
4g 42g 4g

Calories
220
w/applesauce;
300
w/lite
maple syrup

**1 Serving
Equals**
2 Grains
1 Fat

If You Add
These Foods:
2½-3 Fruits
or 1 Fruit
and a 12 oz
Sports Drink

OK To Use For:

PREGAME 2-3 HRS

POST GAME

95

Offside Oatmeal Pancakes

2 egg whites or ¼ cup egg substitute
½ cup all-purpose flour
¾ cup buttermilk
¼ cup skim milk
½ cup quick cooking oats
1 tablespoon sugar
2 tablespoons vegetable oil
½ teaspoon salt (optional)
1 teaspoon baking powder
½ teaspoon baking soda

Blend ingredients together in a bowl. Spray heated non-stick skillet with a vegetable spray. For each pancake, pour ¼ cup batter onto hot skillet. Cook for 2 minutes on first side or until bubbles appear on surface. Flip and cook for another minute, or until heated through. Top each serving with 2 tablespoons maple syrup. (Nutrition values calculated using regular maple syrup, not lite syrup.)

Makes 10 pancakes; serving size 2 pancakes

> **Is your Baking Powder still good?** Test it. Put one half teaspoon baking powder into one quarter cup hot tap water. It should bubble vigorously. If it doesn't, the powder has lost its leavening power and should be thrown away.
>
> **Tip**

All Star Apple-Raisin Breakfast Sandwich

⅓ cup grated apple (red or yellow
   delicious works well)
½ cup fat-free cream cheese, softened
2 tablespoons apple butter
1 teaspoon finely chopped soy nuts
2½ tablespoons smooth peanut butter
⅛ teaspoon cinnamon
12 slices raisin bread, toasted or plain

Grate apples and then pat dry between layers of paper towels (to remove excess moisture). Set aside. Blend cream cheese, apple butter, soy nuts, peanut butter and cinnamon. Then add apple butter and cinnamon. Blend well. Stir in apples.

Spread apple mixture evenly on 6 slices of raisin bread. Place remaining slices on top and cut sandwiches.

Makes 6 sandwiches;
serving size 1 sandwich

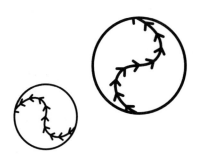

As Is:

POST GAME

Fat Carb Pro
24% 60% 16%
6g   33g   9g

Calories
216

1 Serving Equals
½ Protein
2 Grains
½ Fat

If You Add These Foods:
½ Dairy
3 Fruits or
24 oz Sports
Drink

OK To Use For:

PREGAME 2-3 HRS

POST GAME

As Is:

POST GAME

Fat	Carb	Pro
20%	63%	17%
3g	22g	6g

Calories
282

1 Serving Equals
2 Grains
1 Dairy
1 Fat

If You Add These Foods:
½ Protein
½ Grain
2 Fruits or
12-16 oz
Sports Drink

OK To Use For:

PREGAME 2-3 HRS

POST GAME

Center Court Waffles with Dribble Toppings

WAFFLES
2 cups reduced fat biscuit
     and baking mix
1⅓ cups skim milk
1½ tablespoons vegetable oil
2 egg whites
1 teaspoon vanilla extract

TOPPING
¼ cup of your child's favorite fat-free
     fruit yogurt

Heat waffle iron. Stir ingredients until well blended. Pour mixture onto heated waffle iron (amount depends on your specific iron). Bake until golden brown, about 5 minutes. Carefully remove waffle and top with fat-free yogurt or any of the other suggested toppings listed.

(Nutrition values to your left are for yogurt topping, but all topping suggestions are close in value.)

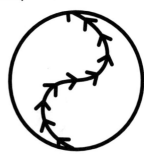

OTHER SUGGESTED TOPPINGS

- Assorted ¼ cup fresh fruit sprinkled with 1 teaspoon powdered sugar (Blueberries, strawberries, red raspberries, grapes, peaches, blackberries, etc.)

- 1 tablespoon cinnamon mixed with ½ cup sugar. Sprinkle 1-2 teaspoons over each warm waffle

- ¼ cup applesauce flavored with cinnamon

- 2 tablespoons maple syrup

Makes 12 waffles (4 inches each); serving size 2 waffles

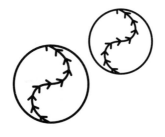

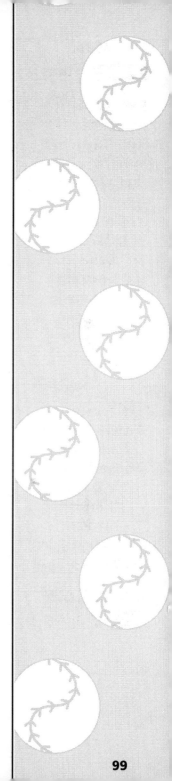

Fat	Carb	Pro
15%	78%	7%
3g	36g	3g

Calories
176

1 Serving
Equals
1-1½ Grains
1 Fruit
½ Fat

If You Add
These Foods:
½ Dairy
1 Fruit

OK To Use For:

PREGAME `1-2 HRS`

POST **GAME**

Banana Wheat Germ MVP Muffins

3 bananas
1¼ cups all-purpose flour
¼ cup wheat germ
2 teaspoons baking powder
1 teaspoon baking soda
¼ teaspoon salt (optional)
⅔ cup sugar
¼-½ teaspoon cinnamon
½ cup raisins (optional)
4 tablespoons extra light margarine,
    room temperature
3 egg whites
1 teaspoon vanilla extract
¼ cup applesauce

Preheat oven to 375 degrees. If you have a food processor: Process bananas with the metal blade until smooth, about 30 seconds. Add remaining ingredients and process for 3-5 seconds. Scrape down the work bowl and process 1 second more.

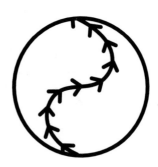

To mix by hand: Mash bananas with fork and set aside. In large mixing bowl, stir all dry ingredients together. Add mashed banana, margarine, egg whites, vanilla extract and applesauce. Stir until all dry ingredients are moistened (lumpy mixture is OK).

Spoon into non-stick, sprayed or greased muffin tins, filling two-thirds full. Bake 15 minutes or until the muffins are golden. Cool in muffin tins for about 8 minutes, then remove to a wire rack.

Makes 12 muffins; serving size 1 muffin

Wheat Germ is a good source of iron, fiber, Vitamins B and E. Wheat germ and whole wheat flour will stay fresher longer if stored in your freezer. Both of these ingredients contain the part of the wheat berry that contains the fat that causes rancidity.

Tip

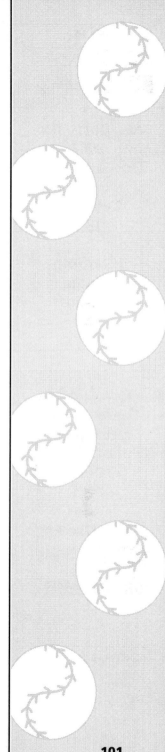

Fat	Carb	Pro
13%	80%	7%
3g	36g	3g

Calories
185

**1 Serving
Equals**
2 Grains

**If You Add
These Foods:**
½-1 Protein
1 Dairy
3 Fruits

OK To Use For:

PREGAME 2-3 HRS

POST GAME

Granola-Almond Marching Muffins

1½ cups reduced fat biscuit
    and baking mix
1 cup firmly packed light brown sugar
1⅛ teaspoons cinnamon
½ cup Craisins (dried cranberries)
1 cup oats
1 cup fat-free honey granola cereal
    with almonds
¾ cup skim milk
1 large egg, slightly beaten
1 tablespoon vegetable oil

Preheat oven to 375 degrees. Blend first three ingredients in a bowl and stir in Craisins, oats and cereal. In a separate bowl, blend milk, egg, and oil. Make a hole in the center of the dry mix and pour in milk mixture. Stir until dry ingredients are moistened (mixture may be lumpy, that's OK). Spoon into non-stick, sprayed or greased muffin tins. Fill three-fourths full. Bake 15-20 minutes or until golden.

Makes 16 muffins; serving size 1 muffin

> The batter for this recipe will be thin. That's the way it's supposed to be. Do not over-stir. If you do, the muffins may turn out tougher than you'd like.
>
> **Tip**

Freestyle Cinnamon Apple Oat Bran Muffins

1 cup all-purpose flour
2 cups whole wheat flour
2½ teaspoons baking soda
1 teaspoon cinnamon
¼ teaspoon nutmeg
1¼ cups oat bran
2 large Rome apples
   (or other cooking apples)
1 can, 12 oz, apple juice concentrate,
   thawed
½ cup water

Preheat oven to 325 degrees. Combine flours with baking soda, cinnamon, and nutmeg. Add oat bran. Peel, core, and coarsely chop the apples and toss with the oat bran mixture. Add the apple juice concentrate and water and mix just until dry ingredients are moistened. Spoon into non-stick, sprayed or greased muffin tins, two-thirds full, and bake for 25 minutes, until golden.

Makes 12 muffins; serving size 1 muffin

Tip

When muffins reach room temperature, place in a plastic bag and freeze for later use.

As Is:

PREGAME	1-2 HRS

POST	GAME

Fat Carb Pro
6%   84%   10%
1g   49g   6g

Calories
210

1 Serving Equals
1½ Grains
1½ Fruits

If You Add These Foods:
1 Dairy
1½ Fruits
1 Fat

OK To Use For:

PREGAME	2-3 HRS

POST	GAME

Fat	Carb	Pro
23%	72%	5%
8g	58g	4g

Calories
315

1 Serving Equals
2½ Grains
1 Fruit
1½ Fats

If You Add These Foods:
1 Protein
2 Grains
1 Dairy
1 Fruit

OK To Use For:

PREGAME 3-4 HRS

POST GAME

Banana Kick Bread

1 stick (½ cup) butter or margarine, room temperature
1½ cups sugar
2 egg whites or ¼ cup egg substitute
3 large bananas, mashed
1 teaspoon vanilla extract
2½ cups all-purpose flour
1 teaspoon baking soda
½ cup raisins or dried fruit (or ½ cup mini chocolate chips)

Preheat oven to 350 degrees. Place butter in mixing bowl. Beat until smooth. Add sugar and blend. Add egg whites. Blend. Add mashed bananas and vanilla. Blend well. Add flour and baking soda, and blend. Stir raisins or dried fruit or chocolate chips into batter. Spray or grease loaf pans, cupcake tins or miniature cupcake tins. Pour batter in loaf pan until it is half filled. Fill cupcake tins until two-thirds full.

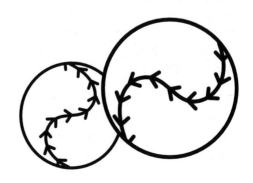

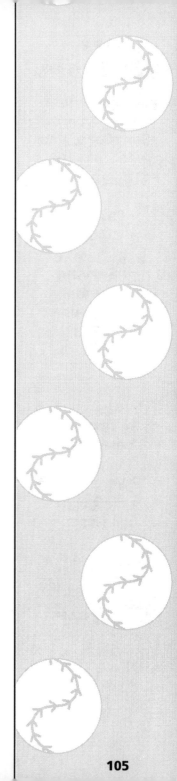

Bake loaf pans for 45 minutes or until toothpick inserted into center comes out clean. Bread should be golden and firm to touch. Bake standard size cupcakes 15-20 minutes. Bake miniature cupcakes about 8-10 minutes. Let muffins cool on a cookie sheet.

This recipe freezes wonderfully. When muffins are cool, transfer to a baggie and freeze.

(Nutrition values calculated with raisins or dried fruit.)

Serves 12; serving size 1 standard muffin, 3 mini muffins

Tip

If your bananas are getting too ripe and you don't have the time to use them, stick them into the freezer (skin and all). On baking day, take the bananas from the freezer and let them thaw a few hours in the refrigerator.

As Is:

PREGAME	2-3 HRS

POST	GAME

Fat	Carb	Pro
25%	70%	6%
11g	72g	6g

Calories
408

1 Serving Equals
4 Grains
2 Fats

If You Add These Foods:
1 Protein
2 Vegetables
½ Dairy
3 Fruits

OK To Use For:

PREGAME	3-4 HRS

POST	GAME

M.C.'s Blueberry Break Coffee Cake

CAKE
¾ cup sugar
2 cups all-purpose flour
2½ teaspoons baking powder
½ teaspoon salt
¼ cup shortening, room temperature
¾ cup skim milk
2 egg whites
2 cups frozen blueberries (thawed and drained) or fresh

CRUMB TOPPING
½ cup sugar
⅓ cup all-purpose flour
¾ teaspoon cinnamon
4 tablespoons margarine

Mix all topping ingredients until crumbly

GLAZE
½ teaspoon vanilla extract
½ cup powdered sugar
1½ to 2 teaspoons hot water

When ready to drizzle on coffee cake, stir all glaze ingredients together

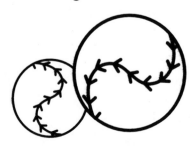

Preheat oven to 375 degrees. Grease or spray a 9 inch square pan or a 9 inch round pan. In electric mixer on medium speed, blend together sugar, flour, baking powder, salt, shortening, milk and egg whites. Beat for 30 seconds. Gently stir in blueberries. Spread batter into prepared pan. Sprinkle with crumb topping. Bake for 45-50 minutes or until a tooth pick inserted into the center comes out clean. Drizzle with glaze. Serve warm.

This is excellent reheated, if there's any left!

Serves 8

Buy extra blueberries when in season and freeze for later use.

Tip

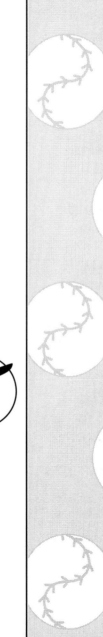

Too High in
Fat and Protein
for Pre-Game.
Not enough
Carbs for
Post-Game

Fat Carb Pro
52% 10% 38%
11g   5g   17g

Calories
186

**1 Serving
Equals**
2½ Proteins
½ Vegetable
1½ Fats

**If You Add
These Foods:**
3 Grains
3 Fruits or
1 Fruit and 16 oz
Sports Drink

OK To Use For:

PREGAME 2-3 HRS

POST GAME

Five-Minute
Free Agent Omelet

1 egg
2 egg whites
2 tablespoons water
¼ cup favorite ingredients, sautéed,
    (listed below)
1 teaspoon olive oil
2 tablespoons favorite low fat cheese
    (listed below)
½ teaspoon garlic powder
¼ teaspoon black pepper
¼ teaspoon dried basil, or 1 teaspoon
    chopped fresh basil
Olive oil vegetable spray

FAVORITE INGREDIENTS: MIX OR MATCH
Chopped red or green pepper, mushrooms, zucchini, fat-free or very lean
turkey bacon or soy sausage.

Sauté above ingredients in 1 teaspoon
olive oil. Drain any liquid before adding
to omelet.

FAVORITE CHEESE:
Shredded low fat mozzarella, cheddar,
low fat Parmesan, or soy "cheese".

Whisk egg, egg whites and water together. Pour ½ of the mixture into a non-stick skillet heated to medium high heat (or spray your pan lightly with olive oil flavored vegetable spray). Cook 1 minute. Sprinkle garlic powder, black pepper and basil over egg. Place sautéed favorite ingredients over omelet. Add cheese. Cook for another minute. With a spatula, gently flip edge of omelet over to meet the opposite edge. Cook 1 more minute. For second omelet, use remaining mixture and repeat process.

Serves 2

To Sauté... cook ingredients quickly in shallow pan with a small amount of oil.

Tip

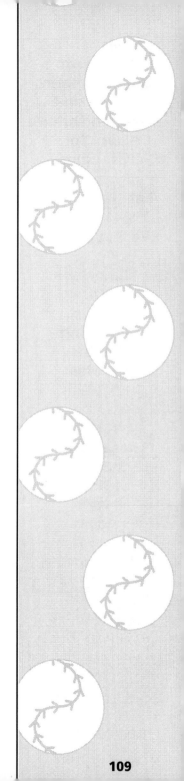

As Is:
Too High in
Fat and Protein
for Pre-Game.
Not enough
Carbs for
Post-Game

Fat	Carb	Pro
26%	40%	34%
7g	26g	22g

Calories
218

**1 Serving
Equals**
1 Protein
1½ Grains

**If You Add
These Foods:**
3 Grains
1 Dairy
3 Fruits
1 Fat

OK To Use For:

PREGAME	3-4 HRS

POST	GAME

Eggs-treme Cheese Burrito

2 cups egg substitute
3 tablespoons skim milk
2 teaspoons light margarine
½ cup low fat cheddar or other
   low fat cheese
4 fat-free tortillas, heated
½ cup salsa

Beat eggs and milk together. Heat margarine in large non-stick skillet. Add egg mixture and cook about 5 minutes, or until eggs are set but still moist. Stir frequently. Stir in cheese. Spoon eggs onto warm tortillas. Top with salsa and roll up.

Try using shredded soy "cheese".
It melts beautifully!

Serves 4

Tip

We're using egg substitute here because egg substitute is lower in fat than eggs. Still, on its own, this recipe is too high in fat and protein to be an ideal Pre-Game selection. But see what happens to the nutritional values (to the left) when we add carbs. This becomes an ideal choice 3-4 hours Pre-Game and for Post-Game.

Half-Time Hot Chocolate

2½ cups instant nonfat dry
    powdered milk
1 cup sugar
1 cup unsweetened cocoa powder
⅛ teaspoon salt
Fat-free whipped topping (optional)

Place dry ingredients in bowl. Whisk or stir until blended. When ready to make a cup of hot chocolate, mix ¼ cup of dry mix and ¾ to 1 cup of boiling water. Top with a tablespoon of fat-free whipped topping, if desired.

Hang-Time Hot Chocolate
Add a teaspoon of cinnamon (or more, to taste) to dry ingredients before mixing.

Makes approximately 18 servings; serving size 1 cup

Make batches of the dry mix ahead and store covered in a cool, dry place.

Tip

As Is:
POST GAME

Fat	Carb	Pro
6%	77%	17%
1g	22g	5g

Calories
104

1 Serving Equals
1 Grain
½ Dairy

If You Add These Foods:
2 Grains

OK To Use For:
PREGAME 1-2 HRS

POST GAME

Chapter Nine
Hand-Off
In A Baggie

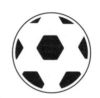

Trish's Switch Hitter Snack Mix

Shot Put Snack Mix

Semi-Pro Snack Mix

Cross Country Trail Mix

Countdown Grand Slam Trail Mix

Goalie Granola

Shane's Tip-Off Taco Munchies

Pop-Up Pizza Popcorn

Championship Chocolate Cherry Brownies

Cherry Pecan Power Bars

Over-The-Limit Oatmeal Treats

Final Four Fruit Cocktail Cookies

Home Run Chocolate Chippers

Honey Bee-Line Cookies

Overtime Chocolate Chip Meringue Cookies

Trish's Switch Hitter Snack Mix

4 cups corn cereal squares
1 cup dry roasted nuts or soy nuts
1 cup raisins
½ cup dried mixed fruit
1 cup yogurt covered raisins
½ cup dried pineapple chunks

Combine all ingredients and store in covered container.

Makes about 16 servings;
serving size ½ cup

Nuts turn rancid when stored at room temperature for extended periods of time. For longer shelf life, put nuts in freezer bags or glass jars and store in freezer.

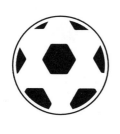

Tip

As Is:

POST GAME

Fat   Carb   Pro
28%   66%   6%
6g   33g   3g

Calories
189

**1 Serving
Equals**
1 Grain
1 Fruit
1 Fat

**If You Add
These Foods:**
1 Protein
4 Grains
2 Vegetables
1 Dairy
1-1½ Fruits

OK To Use For:

PREGAME 3-4 HRS

POST GAME

113

Shot Put Snack Mix

2½ cups mini pretzels, unsalted
1 cup roasted soy nuts
1 cup yogurt covered raisins
½ cup fat-free cheddar cheese cubes

Mix pretzels, soy nuts and raisins.

Store in covered container. Just before serving, add cheese cubes.

Serves 4; serving size 1¼ cup

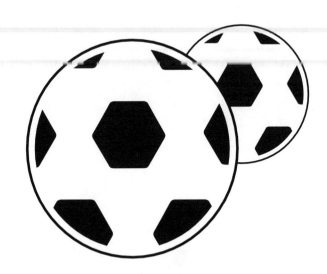

Semi-Pro Snack Mix

½ cup light margarine
1 tablespoon Worcestershire sauce
4 cups corn or rice cereal squares
1 bag microwave low fat popcorn,
    popped (about 5-6 cups popped)
2 cups unsalted mini pretzels

Preheat oven to 250 degrees. Melt margarine and mix with Worcestershire sauce. Place cereal squares in large bowl. Add margarine mixture and stir until well coated. Add popcorn and pretzels. Carefully toss until well mixed. Use a vegetable spray on either a large roasting pan, 15 x 10 x 2 inch, or two smaller pans, or cookie sheets with sides. Bake 1 hour, stirring every 15 minutes from the outside edge into the center because the food around the edges will brown first. Remove from oven and let cool in pan. Transfer to a plastic container and store.

Serves 12; serving size 1 cup

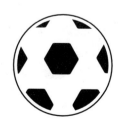

As Is:
Too Low in
Carbs For
Pre and Post
Game

Fat Carb Pro
37% 54% 9%
11g 35g 6g

Calories
233

**1 Serving
Equals**
½ Protein
½ Grain
1 Fruit
2 Fats

**If You Add
These Foods:**
3 Grains
16 oz Sports
Drink

OK To Use For:

PREGAME 2-3 HRS

POST GAME

Cross Country Trail Mix

½ cup mini unsalted pretzels
1 cup dried cherries
1 cup Spanish peanuts, roasted
1 cup banana chips
2 cups plain popped corn

Mix all together. Store in airtight container.

Serves 10; serving size ½ cup

The dried cherries add a bit of sweetness, as do dried cranberries and dried blueberries, which may be used in this recipe instead of cherries.

Tip

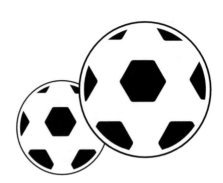

116

Countdown Grand Slam Trail Mix

10 small round Cheerios
 9 pretzel sticks
 8 raisins
 7 fish crackers
 6 chocolate chips
 5 Rice Chex
 4 peanuts
 3 miniature marshmallows
 2 small walnuts, chopped
 1 M & M for good luck!

Place all ingredients in a zip lock bag
and shake.

Serves 1

> Even the littlest tee-ball and
> soccer players can make this
> one all by themselves. The
> counting lesson is a bonus!

Tip

As Is:

POST GAME

Fat	Carb	Pro
27%	66%	8%
5g	28g	3g

Calories
160

**1 Serving
Equals**
1½ Grains
½ Fruit
1 Fat

**If You Add
These Foods:**
1 Protein
2½ Grains
2 Vegetables
1 Dairy
2 Fruits
1½-2 Fats

OK To Use For:

PREGAME **3-4 HRS**

POST GAME

Fat Carb Pro
30% 56% 13%
21g 87g 21g

Calories
293

**1 Serving
Equals**
¾ Protein
1¼ Grains
1 Fruit
1½ Fats

**If You Add
These Foods:**
2 Grains
2 Vegetables
2 Fruits or
1 Fruit and 8 oz
Sports Drink

OK To Use For:

PREGAME **2-3 HRS**

POST GAME

Goalie Granola

6 cups old fashioned rolled oats
½ cup wheat germ (optional)
½ cup sunflower seeds
2 tablespoons honey
2 tablespoons canola oil
2 teaspoons vanilla extract
⅔ cup creamy reduced fat peanut butter
1-1½ cups dried cranberries
¼ cup dried cherries
1½ cups raisins
½ cup soy nuts
½ cup sliced almonds
1 tablespoon cinnamon

Preheat oven to 275 degrees. Combine oats, wheat germ and sunflower seeds in a large bowl. Set aside. Heat honey and oil over medium heat until hot, about one to two minutes. Stir in vanilla and peanut butter and blend until smooth. Pour oil mixture over oat mixture and mix until coated. Use a vegetable spray to coat cookie sheets with sides. Spread mixture evenly onto the cookie sheets and bake approximately 40 minutes. Every 15 minutes stir granola from the outside edge into the center because the granola on the edges will brown first. When the mixture smells fragrant and the oats and sunflower seeds are lightly toasted, the granola is done. Let cool on cookie sheets. Place in large bowl and mix with cranberries, cherries, raisins, soy nuts, almonds and cinnamon. Store in airtight container.

Serves 20; serving size approx. ½ cup

Old fashioned oats, not instant, work better in this recipe because they toast nicely and hold their shape.

Tip

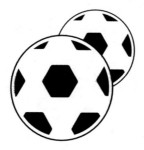

Shane's Tip-Off Taco Munchies

3 cups toasted corn cereal squares
5-6 cups plain popped corn
1 cup mini unsalted pretzels
1 tablespoon taco seasoning
  (or to taste)
3 tablespoons margarine, melted
¼ cup fat-free Parmesan cheese, grated
1 cup fat-free cheddar cheese cubes,
  cut into ¼ inch squares

To Toast Cereal: Preheat oven to 350 degrees. Pour a single layer of cereal squares on baking sheet. Bake for 7-10 minutes, moving the cereal on the outside edges of the baking sheet into the center several times (outside edge cooks faster). When cereal starts to smell fragrant and turns golden, it's done.

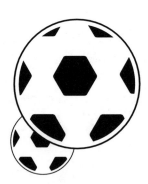

Combine popcorn, cereal and pretzels in a big container. Mix taco seasoning into melted margarine and then drizzle it over popcorn mixture. Sprinkle with Parmesan cheese and toss until coated. Cool. Store in an airtight container. Just before serving, toss with cheddar cheese cubes.

Try substituting Parmesan flavored grated soy "cheese" for regular Parmesan cheese.

Serves l0; serving size 1 cup

When it's your child's turn to take a team snack, try this. Place the dry mix in one container. Put the cheese cubes in a zip lock bag. Right at snack time, toss the cheese cubes in with everything else. (In hot weather, store cheese cubes in an insulated lunch bag.)

Tip

POST GAME

Fat	Carb	Pro
16%	64%	20%
1g	7g	2g

Calories
41

1 Serving Equals
½ Grain

If You Add These Foods:
2 Fruits or 16 oz Sports Drink

OK To Use For:

PREGAME <1 HOUR

POST GAME

Pop-Up Pizza Popcorn

8 cups plain popped corn
Buttery spray (approximately 16 sprays)
½ teaspoon ground dry oregano
½ teaspoon garlic salt
½ teaspoon dry basil
⅛ teaspoon cayenne pepper
¼ cup fat-free grated Parmesan cheese

Spray popped popcorn lightly with buttery spray (approx 16 sprays). Mix spices and cheese together. Sprinkle over popped corn. Toss until coated. Store in airtight container.

Serves 8; serving size 1 cup

Tip

If you like a more spicy taste, add more oregano, salt, basil and cayenne pepper.

Championship Chocolate Cherry Brownies

Cherries or no cherries - you decide
1 cup unsweetened cocoa powder
1 cup flour
Dash of salt
½ teaspoon baking powder
1 cup granulated sugar
1 cup dark brown sugar, packed
1 cup unsweetened applesauce
¼ cup chopped maraschino cherries,
    drained (optional)
2 tablespoons canola oil
1 tablespoon vanilla extract
5 extra large egg whites,
    room temperature

Preheat oven to 350 degrees. Spray a
9 x 13 inch pan with vegetable spray.
Set aside. Stir together cocoa, flour, salt,
baking powder and the two sugars. Set
aside. Blend applesauce, cherries, oil
and vanilla. Pour this applesauce mixture over the cocoa mixture, stirring or
beating until smooth. Set aside. Beat
egg whites until soft peaks form. Then
gently fold into mixture. Pour into pan.
Bake 25-35 minutes, or until toothpick
inserted into center comes out clean.
Don't over bake. Let cool in pan before
cutting into squares.

Makes 24 brownies;
serving size 2 brownies.

As Is:

| PREGAME | <1 HOUR |
| POST | GAME |

Fat	Carb	Pro
9%	83%	7%
2g	39g	3g

Calories
179

1 Serving Equals
2 Grains

If You Add These Foods:
1 Protein
3 Grains
2 Vegetables
1 Dairy
2-2½ Fruits
1 Fat

OK To Use For:

| PREGAME | 3-4 HRS |
| POST | GAME |

Cherry Pecan Power Bars

2 cups quick cooking or instant oatmeal
¾ cup chopped pecans
⅓ cup light stick margarine
½ cup firmly packed dark brown sugar
¼ cup honey
¾ cup dried cherries
¼ cup chopped dried dates
1 cup honey graham cereal squares

Preheat oven to 350 degrees. Pour uncooked oatmeal and chopped pecans onto a cookie sheet with sides. Bake 10 minutes or until golden brown and fragrant (stir every 5 minutes because the mixture on the edges will brown first). When done, set aside. Combine margarine, brown sugar and honey in large saucepan. Cook over medium heat until mixture boils. Pour oat mixture, cherries, dates and cereal squares into honey mixture. Stir until well blended. Coat an 8 inch square baking pan with vegetable

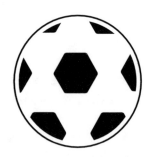

spray and pour in mixture. With lightly floured hands, press firmly into pan. (Note, you may want to wait a bit for the mixture to cool before pressing into pan). Bake for 10-12 minutes. Let cool and cut into 12 bars.

Variations:

Substitute dried cranberries or raisins for the cherries

Serves 12; serving size is 1 bar

Do not use tub margarine in this recipe. Light stick margarine works best.

Tip

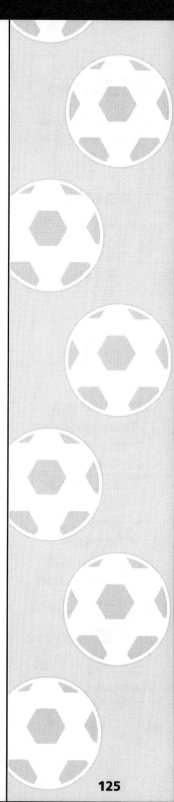

Fat	Carb	Pro
19%	73%	8%
3g	25g	3g

Calories
137

**1 Serving
Equals**
1½ Grains
½ Fat

**If You Add
These Foods:**
½ Protein
2 Grains
2 Vegetables
½ Dairy
2 Fruits
1 Fat
(If you use
variations, do
not add 1 Fat)

OK To Use For:

PREGAME 2-3 HRS

POST GAME

Over-The-Limit
Oatmeal Treats

1 cup granulated sugar
½ cup dark brown sugar, packed
½ cup applesauce
2 extra large eggs
¼ cup canola oil
1¼ teaspoons vanilla extract
2 cups all purpose flour
¾ teaspoon baking powder
¾ teaspoon baking soda
¼ teaspoon salt
1 teaspoon either pumpkin pie spice,
    apple pie spice or cinnamon
3 cups quick rolled oats
1 cup dried cranberries

Preheat oven to 375 degrees. In mixing
bowl (medium speed, if you're using
an electric mixer), beat sugars, applesauce, eggs, oil and vanilla until well
mixed. In separate bowl, blend dry
ingredients and cranberries. Combine
mixtures and blend. (Mixture will be
somewhat sticky but gets less so as it
sits.) On a sprayed or nonstick cookie
sheet, drop dough in rounded tea-
spoonfuls, about 2 inches apart. Bake
8-10 minutes. Don't over bake. Remove
from oven. After cookies cool, store
in airtight container, or freeze.

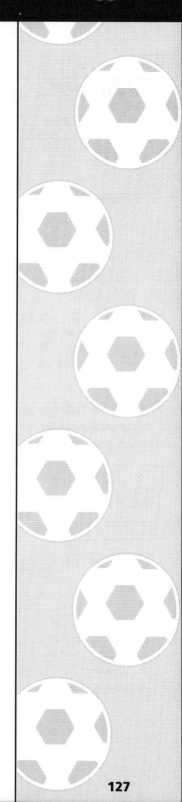

Variations:
- *Chocolate Chip Oatmeal:*
  Add ½ cup mini chocolate chips
- *White Chocolate Chip Oatmeal:*
  add ½ cup white chocolate chips
- *Carob Chip Oatmeal:*
  Add 1 cup carob chips
- *Butterscotch Oatmeal:*
  Add ½ cup butterscotch chips
- *Peanut Butter Oatmeal:*
  Add ½ cup peanut butter chips
- *Caramel Oatmeal:*
  Cut a caramel into 4 pieces and
  push one piece into each cookie
  before baking

With these variations, the fat content
will rise a little, but the cookies will
still fall within the same Pre-Game and
Post-Game categories.

Makes about 5 dozen;
serving size is 2 cookies

Tip

These cookies freeze
very well!

Fat	Carb	Pro
26%	70%	5%
7g	42g	3g

Calories
235

**1 Serving
Equals**
1½ Grains
1 Fruit
1 Fat

**If You Add
These Foods:**
2 Grains
2 Fruits

OK To Use For:

PREGAME 2-3 HRS

POST GAME

Final Four Fruit Cocktail Cookies

½ cup (1 stick) light margarine,
    room temperature
½ cup sugar
½ cup brown sugar, packed
2 egg whites
¾ teaspoon vanilla
1½ cups all-purpose flour
½ teaspoon baking soda
½ teaspoon baking powder
1 teaspoon pumpkin pie spice
¾ – 1 cup fruit cocktail, reduced sugar,
    well drained
1 cup raisins

Preheat oven to 375 degrees. Spray cookie sheets with vegetable spray. Mix margarine with sugar in a large bowl, until creamy. Blend in brown sugar. Add egg whites and vanilla. Beat until mixture is smooth. Set aside. Combine dry ingredients in medium bowl and mix into batter. Stir in fruit cocktail and raisins. Place heaping teaspoons full of batter onto cookie sheets, 2 inches apart. Bake until lightly golden, about 11 to 12 minutes. Transfer to wire cooling racks.

Makes 2 dozen;
serving size is 2 cookies

Home Run Chocolate Chippers

½ cup (1 stick) light margarine, softened
⅓ cup sugar
¾ cup dark brown sugar, packed
2 egg whites
3 tablespoons applesauce
2 teaspoons vanilla extract
1¾ cup all-purpose flour
1 teaspoon baking soda
⅓ cup mini chocolate chips
⅓ cup dried cranberries, raisins or cherries

Preheat oven to 375 degrees. Beat margarine in a mixing bowl on medium speed. Add sugars and egg whites and blend until well mixed. Add applesauce and vanilla and blend. Add dry ingredients and blend again. Finally, mix in chips and berries. Spray cookie sheets with vegetable spray. Place tablespoons full of dough 2 inches apart on sheets. Bake 5 to 7 minutes or until golden brown. Let cool for five minutes and then remove to cooling rack.

Makes 2 dozen cookies; serving size 2 cookies

As Is:

POST GAME

Fat	Carb	Pro
18%	76%	5%
4g	41g	3g

Calories
210

1 Serving Equals
2 Grains
1 Fat

If You Add These Foods:
½-1 Protein
½ Grain
2-2½ Vegetables
1 Dairy
1 Fruit

OK To Use For:

PREGAME 2-3 HRS

POST GAME

As Is:

POST GAME

Fat	Carb	Pro
24%	71%	5%
5g	33g	2g

Calories
177

1 Serving Equals
2 Grains
1 Fat

If You Add These Foods:
½-1 Protein
1 Grain
2-2½ Vegetables
1 Dairy
1 Fruit

OK To Use For:

PREGAME 2-3 HRS

POST GAME

Honey Bee-Line Cookies

½ cup (1 stick) light margarine
2 egg whites
½ cup honey
½ cup brown sugar, packed
1½ cups all-purpose flour
¼ teaspoon salt
½ teaspoon baking soda
¾ teaspoon ground cinnamon

Preheat oven to 375 degrees. Beat margarine, egg whites, honey and brown sugar in a medium bowl. Scrape bowl frequently until mixture is smooth. Stir in all remaining ingredients. Place teaspoons full of dough onto ungreased cookie sheet, 1 inch apart. Bake until light brown, about 7 to 9 minutes. Remove from oven. Leave on cookie sheet for 3 to 5 minutes before moving cookies to cooling racks.

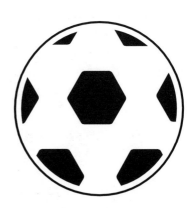

Variations:
- *Honey-Raisin:*
  Add ½ cup raisins to the batter
- *Honey-Cinnamon:*
  Mix ⅔ teaspoon cinnamon with 2 tablespoons of sugar. Sprinkle on cookies after removing them from the oven
- *Honey-Coconut:*
  Add ¾ cup shredded coconut to the batter
- *Honey-Bran:*
  Add ¾ cup shredded bran cereal to the batter

With these variations, the calories and the carbohydrates will go up a little. But the cookies will still fall within the same Pre-Game, Post-Game categories.

Makes 2 dozen cookies; serving size 2 cookies

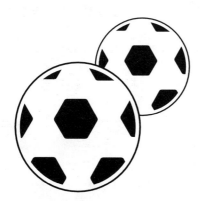

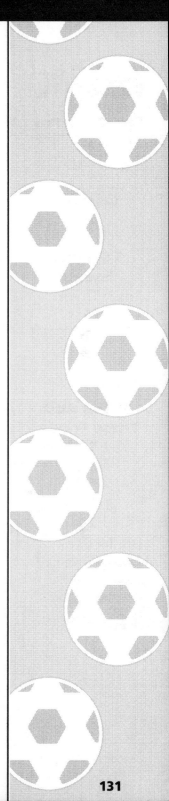

As Is:

POST GAME

Fat	Carb	Pro
17%	78%	4%
4g	42g	2g

Calories
206

1 Serving Equals
2½ Grains
½ Fat

___

If You Add These Foods:
½-1 Protein
2-2½ Vegetables
1 Dairy
3 Fruits

OK To Use For:

PREGAME 2-3 HRS

POST GAME

Overtime Chocolate Chip Meringue Cookies

3 egg whites from large eggs,
    room temperature
1 teaspoon vanilla extract
Dash of salt
¼ teaspoon cream of tartar
1 cup sugar
½ cup mini semi-sweet chocolate chips

Preheat oven to 275 degrees. Place room temperature egg whites, vanilla, dash of salt, and cream of tartar in electric mixing bowl. Beat until soft peaks form. Gradually add the sugar and continue beating until stiff peaks form. Now you have meringue! Fold in chocolate chips. Cover a 9 x 12 inch cookie sheet with plain ungreased brown paper (you can use a lunch bag). Using a tablespoon, scoop out a generous helping of meringue and place on the brown paper, space 1 inch apart. Continue until all of the meringue is gone. Place on the middle rack of the oven and bake for 1 hour.

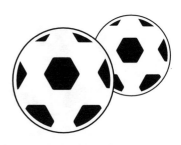

At 1 hour, turn oven off and let cookies dry in the oven with the door closed for an additional 2 hours. Store in an airtight container.

Makes 12 cookies; serving size 2 cookies

Tip

While these cookies are easy to make, they do require a little "overtime" from the baker. A time saving tip...if you're using more than 1 cookie tray, place second tray on the top shelf of the oven and switch trays halfway through both the baking process and the cooling process.

Chapter Ten

"Checking" In The Cooler

Bella's Chocolate Rebound Bars

Chocolate Mousse Pudding Play

Sudden Death Chocolate Fruit Tips

Paige's Vanilla-Chocolate Chip Power Pudding

Hole-In-One-Granola Parfaits

Mary's Home Plate Yogurt

Sideline Sun-Cooked Fruit Leather

Home Court Chunky Applesauce

Annamarie's Major League Lemon Squares

Old-Timer's Orange Cubes

Base Hit Banana Popsicles

Pink Lemonade Dream Team-Sicles

Peanut Butter Puck Ice Cream Sandwiches

Bella's Chocolate Rebound Bars

½ cup sugar
½ cup unsweetened cocoa
2½ cups 1% milk or skim milk
1 teaspoon chocolate syrup
1 teaspoon vanilla extract

In a medium saucepan, blend together the sugar and cocoa. Stir in the milk and cook over medium-low heat. Stir to dissolve the sugar and cocoa, until bubbles appear, but do not allow to boil. Remove from the heat. Add the syrup and vanilla. Stir well. Pour mixture into 4 ice pop containers with sticks, or into paper cups (add sticks when partially frozen). Freeze until frozen, about 3-4 hours.

Serves 4; serving size 1 pop

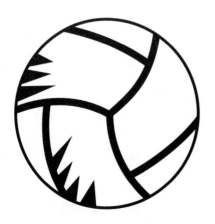

As Is:

PREGAME	<1 HOUR
POST	GAME

Fat Carb Pro
13% 74% 13%
3g 39g 7g

Calories
190

1 Serving Equals
1½ Grains
1 Dairy

If You Add These Foods:
1 Fruit
or 8 oz
Sports Drink

OK To Use For:

PREGAME	1-2 HRS
POST	GAME

PREGAME <1 HOUR

POST GAME

Fat	Carb	Pro
8%	84%	9%
1g	24g	3g

Calories
116

**1 Serving
Equals**
½ Grain
1 Vegetable
½ Fat

**If You Add
These Foods:**
⅓ Protein
1 Grain
1 Fruit

OK To Use For:

PREGAME 1-2 HRS

POST GAME

Chocolate Mousse Pudding Play

1⅓ cups low fat soy milk,
    vanilla flavored
1 tablespoon nonfat dry milk
1 box, 1.4 oz, instant sugar free,
    fat-free chocolate pudding mix
1 cup fat-free whipped topping

Blend soy and dry milk together. Add pudding mix. Whisk until blended. Fold in whipped topping, blending well. Spoon into glasses. Place in refrigerator until set (about 30 minutes).

Variations:
Pistachio Cream: A tropical treat! Follow instructions above, except use sugar free, fat-free instant pistachio pudding. Fold in 1 cup crushed unsweetened pineapple (drained), before folding in whipped topping. (Nutrition values are very close to what you'll see in the bar to your left)

Crunchy Banana: It's like old-fashioned banana pudding! Follow instructions above except use sugar free instant vanilla pudding. Add 1 teaspoon vanilla to the soy milk, and blend in 1 chopped banana. Then fold in whipped topping. Top with 6 low fat vanilla wafers, crumbled. (Nutrition values are very close to what you'll see in the bar to your left)

Chocolate Peanut Butter: Follow instructions above except blend in ¼ cup reduced fat peanut butter before folding in whipped topping. (OK **As Is**: Pre-Game 2-3 hours and Post-Game)

Double Chocolate Rocky Road: Follow instructions above except fold in ¼ cup chopped nuts and 2 tablespoons miniature chocolate chips before folding in whipped topping. (OK **As Is**: Pre-Game 2-3 hours and Post-Game)

Serves 4; serving size ¾ cup

You may use skim milk instead of soy milk. But try making this recipe at least once with soy milk, for that extra boost of nutrition. The soy really makes the chocolate flavor "jump out"!

Tip

As Is:

POST GAME

Fat	Carb	Pro
26%	70%	4%
4g	27g	2g

Calories
144

1 Serving
Equals
½ Grain
1 Fruit
½ Fat

If You Add
These Foods:
1 Protein
3½ Grains
2 Vegetables
1 Dairy
3 Fruits
½ Fat

OK To Use For:

PREGAME 3-4 HRS

POST GAME

Sudden Death Chocolate Fruit Tips

Think of the chocolate here as icing on just the very tip of the fruit. This may be a way to get your child to eat a fresh strawberry!

8 oz (approx) semi-sweet chocolate, melted
1 quart of large strawberries, or
2 medium bananas (cut into 1 inch chunks), or
½ lb (approx) of dried apricots or banana chips (Use plain banana chips, dried without oil, sugar or honey. You may have to visit a health food store to find these.)

Melt semi-sweet chocolate in microwave on medium heat for about 2 minutes, or until mixture is mostly melted but lumpy. Remove and stir until smooth. (To melt on your stove, use a nonstick saucepan or double boiler.) Dip each piece of fruit into melted chocolate, covering just the tip (about a quarter of the way up) with a thin coat. (The more the chocolate, the greater the percentage of fat.) Then, lay each piece of tipped fruit on a vegetable sprayed piece of foil (or wax paper) on a tray. If using fresh strawberries, wash and dry them well, leaving the stem on for easy dipping.

Place in refrigerator to harden. Store in refrigerator, covered.

Serves 4 or more;
serving size 4 pieces of fruit

Tip

It's hard to measure accurately here, because the fruit you use will be different sizes. So, be prepared to use a little more chocolate, if absolutely needed. Stick with 4 pieces of tipped fruit per serving and you should stay within our Pre and Post-Game Guidelines.

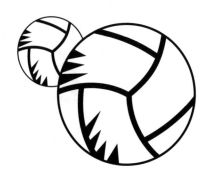

Fat	Carb	Pro
15%	77%	8%
3g	40g	4g

Calories
194

1 Serving Equals
2 Grains
½ Dairy
½ Fat

If You Add These Foods:
½-1 Protein
1 Grain
2-2½ Vegetables
½ Dairy
2 Fruits

OK To Use For:

PREGAME 2-3 HRS

POST GAME

Paige's Touchdown Vanilla-Chocolate Chip Pudding

½ cup sugar
⅛ teaspoon salt
2 tablespoons cornstarch
1½ cups plain soy milk
1 teaspoon vanilla extract
4 tablespoons mini chocolate chips

In a medium-sized saucepan, before putting over heat, stir together sugar, salt, and cornstarch. Slowly add the soy milk, stirring constantly to prevent lumps. Then, over medium heat, bring mixture to a boil. Lower heat to simmer, stirring constantly for about 5 minutes. Mixture should now be thick and creamy. Remove from the stove and stir in vanilla. Cool until lukewarm. Add chocolate chips and stir. Pour into cups. Refrigerate until mixture sets, about 30-45 minutes.

Serves 4; serving size ½ cup

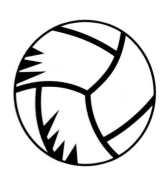

Hole-In-One Granola Parfait

¼ cup nonfat granola
1 cup low fat yogurt, any flavor
½ cup fresh or frozen berries or
    diced fruit of your choice

In a glass, layer all ingredients: granola on bottom, then yogurt, then fruit.

If the parfait is going to the game in a cooler, use a plastic container with a cover (single serving size). The ingredients may be a bit "in the rough" by the time the Hole-In-One Parfait is served, but we promise it will still taste just as good.

Serves 1

Tip

Lemon yogurt is a good match with frozen or fresh berries.

As Is:

PREGAME	1-2 HRS
POST	GAME

Fat	Carb	Pro
13%	69%	18%
5g	58g	15g

Calories
321

1 Serving Equals
3½ Grains
½ Fruit
½ Fat

If You Add These Foods:
½ Protein
1 Dairy
2-2½ Vegetables
1 Fruit

OK To Use For:

PREGAME	2-3 HRS
POST	GAME

Fat	Carb	Pro
5%	61%	34%
3g	18g	10g

Calories
118

1 Serving Equals
1 Dairy

If You Add These Foods:
1 Protein
4 Grains
2 Vegetables
2-2½ Fruits
1 Fat

OK To Use For:

PREGAME 3-4 HRS

POST GAME

Mary's Home Plate Yogurt

3½ cups skim milk
⅓ cup nonfat dry milk powder
4 tablespoons plain low fat yogurt,
      room temperature

In heavy saucepan, combine milk and dry milk. Over low heat, stirring frequently, heat milk until steam rises and milk is scalded (tiny bubbles will appear around the edges of the pan, and milk will reach a temperature of 160 degrees). Remove from heat and cover loosely. Cool until lukewarm (about 98 degrees). Whisk in yogurt. Transfer to covered container. Let container rest in a "warm place", undisturbed for 6-10 hours, or until thickened.

Examples of "warm places"...
1. Rita wraps her covered container completely in a thick towel and leaves it undisturbed on the counter
2. Leave the container in a turned-off gas oven. The pilot light will give off enough heat to do the trick
3. Fill a small cooler with warm tap water, about halfway up, and set sealed container inside

What will happen during this time is that the yogurt cultures will activate in the milk, turning the mixture into home-made yogurt. Store in refrigerator.

Serves 4; serving size 1 cup

Typically, homemade yogurt is not as thick as commercial yogurt, but we think homemade yogurt tastes better! Make your own fruit fla-vored yogurt by stirring in 1 table-spoon of all-fruit jam or preserves (1 table-spoon per cup).

Tip

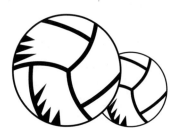

As Is:

PREGAME <1 HOUR

POST GAME

Fat Carb Pro
4%   95%   1%
0g   29g   0g

Calories
112

**1 Serving
Equals**
1½ Fruits

**If You Add
These Foods:**
⅓ Protein
2 Grains

OK To Use For:

PREGAME 1-2 HRS

POST GAME

Sideline Sun-Cooked Fruit Leather

5 pounds apples or pears
½-1 cup water or ½ cup apple juice
½ cup sugar (optional)
1-2 teaspoons cinnamon (optional)

There are four steps to this recipe: Preparation, Cooking, Puréeing and Drying

Preparation
Wash, core and cut fruit into chunks

Cooking Options
• *Crock Pot or Slow Cooker Method:* Spray the crock pot with a non-stick vegetable spray. Place fruit in crock pot and add ½ cup water or ½ cup apple juice (use apple juice with pears, too). Cook on low, 8 to 10 hours
• *Stovetop Method:* Place in a heavy or nonstick pot. Add 1 cup water or ½ cup water and ½ cup apple juice. Simmer until fruit is soft enough to mash with a fork. If mixture starts to stick, add additional water

Purée
After fruit is cooked, run mixture through either a food mill or sieve, or use a blender or food processor.
    If desired, use ½ cup sugar to sweeten. Stir sugar and/or cinnamon into mashed fruit while it's still warm.

Drying Options

- *To Dry in the Sun:* The heat from summer's sun will evaporate the moisture from the fruit, turning it into a sheet of leather. Cover cookie sheets (with sides) with foil. Spray foil with vegetable spray. Spread fruit mixture on foil, about ¼ inch thick. Cover with cheesecloth or netting to keep dust and insects out. Place outside in sun. Bring in at night or if it rains. It will take from 2 days to a week for the fruit purée to dry, depending upon the weather. You'll know it's ready when the moisture has evaporated and the leather has shrunk, and you are left with a thin sheet of leather that can be pulled right up off the foil.
- *To Dry in the Oven:* Dry in warm oven, up to 120 degrees. Leave oven door open slightly so moisture can escape. Leather will be ready in 4 to 6 hours, or when mixture can be pulled away easily from the foil in a thin sheet. Let cool to room temperature.

To store, lay fruit leather flat on plastic wrap or foil and roll up. Store in airtight container away from heat and light. Keeps at room temperature for up to two months. Lasts up to 6 months in refrigerator, and up to 1 year stored in freezer.

(Our nutrition values were calculated using ½ cup apple juice and ½ cup sugar.)

Serves 16; serving size is approx. 1½ inches wide by 15 inches long

> **Tip**
>
> Don't peel that apple! Much of an apple's healing power is in the skin, which contains super antioxidants—To remove any toxins or pesticides naturally, put 2 cups cider vinegar into a kitchen sink full of lukewarm water. Add unpeeled fruit. Take a washcloth and gently scrub fruit. Rinse in clear water. Dry before using.

145

PREGAME <1 HOUR
POST GAME

Fat	Carb	Pro
4%	95%	1%
0g	31g	0g

Calories
119

**1 Serving
Equals**
1½ Fruits

**If You Add
These Foods:**
1 Grain
½ Dairy

OK To Use For:

PREGAME 1-2 HRS
POST GAME

Home Court
Chunky Applesauce

5 pounds apples
½ cup apple juice or as much water
    as needed
½ cup sugar and cinnamon (optional)

Wash, core and cut apples into chunks.
Leave the skin on for more nutrition
and taste. (See previous recipe for
tip on how to remove pesticides from
fruit naturally.)

Cooking Options
Crock Pot or Slow Cooker Method:
Place in sprayed crock pot and add
½ cup apple juice or water. Cook on
low, 8 to 10 hours, or until very soft.

Stovetop Method: Use a heavy, large
pot because mixture tends to "sputter"
when it cooks. Start out adding 4 cups
water, or 3½ cups water and ½ cup
apple juice. Bring to a boil and lower
to a simmer. If mixture starts to stick,
add more water, starting with ½ cup.
Mixture should be thick. Cook until
mixture is very soft.

If desired, after mixture has cooked and is still warm, add sugar and cinnamon, to taste. For a smoother applesauce, run mixture through food mill, blender, or food processor.

Let cool and store in refrigerator. Makes about 2 quarts, depending upon apples used. (May also be made with pears. Follow same instructions.)

(Our nutrition values were calculated using ½ cup apple juice and ½ cup sugar.)

Serves 16; serving size is about ½ cup

If you want the sauce to stay snowy white, sprinkle on some commercial fruit preserver (called "Fruit Fresh") right after you cut the fruit into chunks. Or, place the apple or pear chunks into a bowl of water and lemon juice (use juice of 1 lemon).

Tip

As Is:

POST GAME

Fat Carb Pro
23% 70% 7%
6g   42g   4g

Calories
234

1 Serving Equals
2½ Grains
1 Fat

___

If You Add These Foods:
½-1 Protein
1 Grain
2-2½ Vegetables
1 Dairy
1 Fruit

OK To Use For:

PREGAME 2-3 HRS

POST GAME

Annamarie's Major League Lemon Squares

CRUST:
1 cup sifted all-purpose flour
¼ cup confectioner sugar
¼ cup fat-free cream cheese, room temperature
3 tablespoons canola oil

FILLING:
1 egg
2 egg whites
1 cup sugar
2 tablespoons fresh lemon juice
½ teaspoon baking powder
¼ teaspoon salt

Preheat oven to 350 degrees. Spray an 8 inch baking pan with vegetable spray. To make crust, blend flour, sugar, cream cheese and canola oil. Press into bottom and ½ inch up sides of pan. Bake 20 minutes.

While crust is baking, use mixer to blend egg and egg whites. Then add sugar and mix well. Add lemon juice, baking powder and salt, and continue blending. Pour into baked crust and bake an additional 25 minutes, or until slightly golden in color. Cool before serving. Keep refrigerated. You can lightly sift powdered sugar on top, if desired.

Serves 8; serving size 2 inch square

Old-Timer's Orange Cubes

1 dozen oranges-halved

Wash and dry several plastic ice cube trays. Either by hand or with an electric juicer, squeeze juice from oranges and pour into prepared trays (be sure to remove any seeds). Freeze. Pop cubes out individually. Eat with a fork or fingers.

Serving size 4 cubes

> Be creative and freeze other healthy juices: apple, cranberry, pineapple, guava, or grape. It's also fun to serve juice cubes in a lemon or lime beverage.

Tip

As Is:

PREGAME	<1 HOUR
POST	GAME

Fat	Carb	Pro
4%	90%	6%
0g	12g	0g

Calories
60

1 Serving Equals
1 Fruit

If You Add These Foods:
1/3 Protein
2 Grains

OK To Use For:

PREGAME	1-2 HRS
POST	GAME

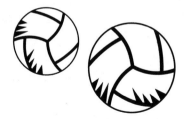

Fat Carb Pro
15% 77% 9%
4g 50g 6g

Calories
246

1 Serving Equals
1½ Grains
1½ Fruits
½ Fat

If You Add These Foods:
½-1 Protein
½-1 Grain
2-2½ Vegetables
1 Dairy

OK To Use For:

| PREGAME | 2-3 HRS |

| POST | GAME |

Base Hit Banana Popsicles

½ cup vanilla yogurt
1 tablespoon peanut butter
1-2 teaspoons sugar
1 cup low fat granola cereal, crushed
4 small bananas

Combine yogurt, peanut butter, and sugar. Cut four large squares of plastic wrap. Pour ¼ cup cereal on each square. Peel bananas and insert 1 popsicle stick into each. Coat bananas with yogurt mixture and then roll the banana in cereal until coated evenly. Then wrap it all up in the plastic. Twist ends to hold everything in. Freeze or refrigerate until ready to eat.

Serves 4; serving size 1 banana

> To keep bananas longer, refrigerate with the peel left on. The peel will turn black but banana will be OK.
>
> **Tip**

Pink Lemonade Dream-Teamsicles

1 pint plain fat-free yogurt
6-8 tablespoons frozen pink lemonade
   concentrate, thawed
1 teaspoon vanilla extract

Blend all ingredients together well. Pour into four 6 oz paper cups. When partially frozen, insert popsicle sticks.

Orange Dream-Teamsicles

Follow instructions above but substitute 6-8 tablespoons frozen orange juice concentrate, thawed, and $\frac{1}{2}$ teaspoon orange zest (grated orange peel), optional.

Makes 6-8 popsicles;
serving size 1 popsicle

> **Tip**
> If you're going to serve these right from the cooler at the ball field, skip the popsicle sticks and pack plastic spoons instead.

As Is:

POST GAME

Fat	Carb	Pro
2%	74%	24%
0g	22g	7g

Calories
118

1 Serving Equals
1 Grain
1 Dairy

If You Add These Foods:
$\frac{1}{2}$-1 Protein
2 Grains
2-2$\frac{1}{2}$ Vegetables
1 Fruit

OK To Use For:

PREGAME 2-3 HRS

POST GAME

151

Calories
274

1 Serving Equals
½ Protein
2½ Grains
½ Fruit
1 Fat

If You Add These Foods:
½ Protein
2 Grains
2 Vegetables
1 Dairy
2 Fruits

OK To Use For:

PREGAME 3-4 HRS

POST GAME

Peanut Butter Puck Ice Cream Sandwiches

⅓ cup firmly packed light brown sugar
¼ cup 1% milk
⅓ cup reduced fat chunky peanut butter
2 large egg whites
½ cup quick cooking or instant oats
⅓ cup unsifted all-purpose flour
¼ teaspoon salt
¼ teaspoon baking soda
⅓ cup chopped pitted dates
4 cups low fat frozen vanilla yogurt
¼ cup chocolate chips, melted

Using a food processor and the steel blade, combine brown sugar, milk, peanut butter and egg whites. Process until blended. In a separate bowl, combine oats, flour, salt, and baking soda. Add this mixture to peanut butter mixture in processor. Pulse until all ingredients are well mixed.

Stir in dates. Lightly spray an 8 inch square glass or microwave-safe baking dish with vegetable spray. Spread mixture evenly into the dish. Microwave on medium (50 percent power), 6 to 7 minutes or until cake tester inserted into center comes out clean and top is mostly dry. Cool to room temperature.

When cool, cut into eight 4 inch squares. Slice each in half. Spread ¼ cup softened ice cream on bottom half. Put other half on top to make sandwich. Freeze until firm. When ready to serve, melt chocolate in microwave in a microwave-safe bowl on medium power, about one and a half minutes. Some small lumps will remain. Remove from microwave and stir until smooth. Take ice cream sandwiches from freezer and drizzle melted chocolate on top of each sandwich. Refreeze sandwiches until chocolate is firm, about 5 minutes.

Serves 8; serving size 1 sandwich

Tip

To transport in a cooler (with several ice packs), wrap each ice cream sandwich individually in foil and then place each in a plastic sandwich bag.

Chapter Eleven
Point Spreads

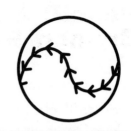

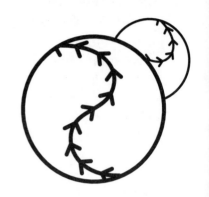

Peanut Butter Crunch Break

Free Style Herb Spread

Volley Veggie Wrap

Drop Kick Deli Wrap

Nutty Break-Away Graham Crackers

Cheddar Cheese Tofu Touchdown

Rice Cake Rush

Superbowl Vegetables and Dip

Backcourt Bagel Bites

Two-on-Two Tuna Spread

Chunky Salsa Chip Shot

Ace Cinnamon Spread

Fruit Be Forehand

Coach Eda's Winning Whipped Delight

Peanut Butter Crunch Break

1 cup reduced fat peanut butter
½ cup shredded carrot
2 tablespoons shelled sunflower seeds
¼ cup raisins
3 tablespoons honey

Mix all ingredients together well.
Cover and refrigerate.

Serve on vegetables, fruit or on low fat crackers. (We calculated 5 crackers per serving in our nutrition values.)

Makes 2 cups, 32 servings; serving size 1 tablespoon

Tip

Peanut butter is a great quick source of carbohy-drates, protein, folate and Vitamin E. Although peanut butter is high in fat, it doesn't take much to turn it into a balanced snack. Just add some crackers or whole wheat bread, plus a sports bever-age or a piece of fruit and you have a nutritionally well-rounded snack.

As Is:

POST GAME

Fat	Carb	Pro
25%	61%	14%
6g	35g	7g

Calories
219

1 Serving Equals
½ Protein
1½ Grains
1 Fat

If You Add These Foods:
0-½ Protein
2 Grains
2 Vegetables
1 Dairy
1 Fruit

OK To Use For:

PREGAME 3-4 HRS

POST GAME

155

POST GAME

Fat	Carb	Pro
6%	65%	28%
0g	12g	5g

Calories
66

1 Serving Equals
½ Protein
1½ Vegetables

If You Add These Foods:
3 Fruits or
1 Fruit
and 16 oz
Sports Drink

OK To Use For:

PREGAME 1-2 HRS

POST GAME

Free Style Herb Spread

1 pkg., 8 oz, fat-free cream cheese, softened
4 oz low fat silken tofu, drained
½ oz, ½ pkg. or less, dry powdered ranch dressing mix

Blend all ingredients well. Cover and refrigerate.

Use this herb spread to stuff celery, spread on low fat crackers, or as a "dunk" for fresh veggies. (In our nutrition values we calculated 3 celery ribs, about 3 inches each, per serving.)

Makes 1½ cups, 24 servings; serving size 1 tablespoon

> **Tip**
> Since powdered ranch dressing mixes tend to be strongly flavored, start out using less rather than more and adjust to taste. To add crunch, color and more vitamins, toss in a handful of shredded carrots.

Volley Veggie Wrap

1 flour tortilla, fat-free (about 10")
2 tablespoons light shredded
    cheddar cheese
½ cup cut veggies from salad bar
    or home
2 tablespoons favorite light salad
    dressing

Layer veggies and cheese on tortilla.
Top with dressing. Roll up.

Serves 1

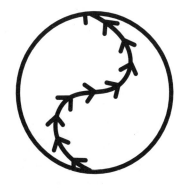

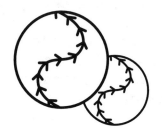

As Is:

PREGAME 1-2 HRS

POST GAME

Fat	Carb	Pro
15%	68%	16%
4g	50g	13g

Calories
294

1 Serving
Equals
½ Protein
3 Grains
½ Vegetable
1 Fat

If You Add
These Foods:
0-½ Protein
1½-2 Vegetables
1 Dairy
1 Fruit

OK To Use For:

PREGAME 2-3 HRS

POST GAME

As Is:

POST GAME

Fat	Carb	Pro
17%	57%	26%
8g	62g	28g

Calories
425

**1 Serving
Equals**
1 Protein
3 Grains
1½ Fats

**If You Add
These Foods:**
20 oz Sports
Drink
or
2½ Fruits

OK To Use For:

PREGAME 2-3 HRS

POST GAME

Drop Kick Deli Wrap

1 flour tortilla, fat-free (about 10")
2 tablespoons light or fat-free
    mayonnaise
3 oz thin sliced deli turkey or roast
    beef
1 oz low fat cheese
2 tablespoons shredded carrots

Spread mayonnaise on tortilla. Layer
turkey, cheese and carrot on top. Roll up.

Serves 1

For a Deli-Wrap with "Chili" Mayo,
add a dash of chili powder to mayonnaise and blend well. For
"Horseradish" Mayo, add
horseradish, to taste, and
blend well.

Tip

Nutty Break-Away Graham Crackers

1 box of your favorite plain graham crackers
1 tablespoon reduced fat peanut butter
3 tablespoons raisins
2 tablespoons soy nuts, chopped

Break 2 whole graham crackers in half, giving you 4 separate and equal squares. Spread 1 tablespoon of peanut butter on 2 of the 4 crackers. Place raisins and soy nuts on top of the peanut butter. Cover each prepared cracker with the 2 remaining graham crackers.

Variations
- Try thin apple slices on the peanut butter.
- Use apple butter instead of peanut butter.
- Spread low fat cream cheese on graham crackers and add raisins.

(Our nutrition values are based on the top recipe.)

Serves 1

Experiment with other healthy nuts and with seeds: sunflower, pumpkin, or sesame.

Tip

As Is:
POST GAME

Fat	Carb	Pro
25%	65%	10%
9g	52g	8g

Calories
302

1 Serving Equals
1½ Proteins
1½ Grains
1½ Fruits
2 Fats

If You Add These Foods:
2 Grains
2-2½ Vegetables
½ Dairy

OK To Use For:
PREGAME 2-3 HRS
POST GAME

POST	GAME

Fat	Carb	Pro
30%	65%	5%
6g	32g	3g

Calories
200

1 Serving
Equals
2 Grains
½ Vegetable
1 Fat

If You Add
These Foods:
1 Protein
2 Grains
1 Dairy
3 Fruits

OK to Use For:

PREGAME	3-4 HRS

POST	GAME

Cheddar Cheese Tofu Touchdown

2 low fat cheddar cheese flavored
    rice cakes
2 tofu "Veggie Slices", Cheddar Flavor
    (a cheese alternative made with tofu)
2 tablespoons any of the following:
    chopped green jalapenos or canned
        green chilies
    shredded carrot
    chopped green onions
    chopped bell pepper
    chopped tomatoes

Put one Veggie Slice (1 slice is ¾ oz) on each rice cake. If desired, top with 2 tablespoons of chopped vegetables. Microwave on high for 30 seconds, or until the Veggie Slices turn into a creamy, cheesy sauce.

Variations
Veggie Slices come in other flavors: Swiss, Provolone and Pepper Jack

Serving size 2 rice cakes w/toppings

Rice Cake Rush

2 of your child's favorite rice cakes
1 tablespoon reduced fat
    peanut butter or
1 tablespoon reduced fat
    cream cheese or
1 tablespoon shredded cheddar,
    farmer, or mozzarella cheese

Place 2 rice cakes on a plate. Top with 1 tablespoon of peanut butter, or 1 tablespoon of cream cheese, or 1 table-spoon of shredded cheese.

Serving size 2 rice cakes w/topping

Calories will change somewhat depending on which topping used. Other nutritional values will remain within the same Pre and Post-Game ranges.

These travel well to school or to the game on a paper plate loosely covered with foil.

Tip

As Is:
Too High in Fat and Low in Carbs for Pre and Post-Game

Fat Carb Pro
42% 41% 17%
12g   26g   10g

Calories
230
w/peanut butter;
140
w/cream cheese;
120
w/cheddar cheese

1 Serving Equals
1 Protein
1 Grain
2 Fats

If You Add These Foods:
2 Grains
2 Fruits

OK To Use For:

| PREGAME | 2-3 HRS |
| POST | GAME |

161

As Is:
Too High in Fat
and Too Low
in Carbs
for Pre or
Post-Game

Fat	Carb	Pro
50%	41%	9%
7g	13g	3g

Calories
128

1 Serving Equals
2 Vegetables
1½ Fats

If You Add These Foods:
4 Grains
1 Dairy
1 Fruit

PREGAME 2-3 HRS

POST GAME
OK To Use For:

Superbowl Veggies and Dip

Choose from a variety of vegetables
you know your child will like.
Here are a few suggestions:
  miniature carrots
  red or green pepper cut into strips
  sugar snap peas
  broccoli or cauliflower florets
  cucumbers, peeled and sliced
  blanched, chilled green beans
  blanched, chilled asparagus
  mushrooms
2 tablespoons light ranch dressing

Quick and Easy Method
Purchase a jar of low fat ranch dressing. Put two tablespoons of dressing
on your child's plate and let the dipping begin.

Serving size 1 cup vegetables and 2
tablespoons light dressing

Do you have a picky-eater who
turns up his or her nose whenever
you try to introduce a new food?
Studies show it may take 8 to10
exposures to a new food before
a child will actually like it.
So don't give up easily!

Tip

Backcourt Bagel Bites

½ plain sliced bagel or ½ raisin bagel
   (½ of a 3 oz bagel), and either

1 tablespoon reduced fat peanut
   butter with
¼ medium apple, sliced thinly

   or

1 tablespoon reduced fat
   cream cheese with
2 tablespoons shredded carrots

On a toasted ½ bagel, put peanut butter and sliced apple, or cream cheese
and shredded carrot.

Serves 1

**For convenience, you may
purchase sliced plain bagels
in your grocer's freezer case,
or buy fresh bagels from your
favorite bagel store or bakery. Slice
and store fresh bagels in zip lock
freezer bags in freezer for later use.**

Tip

As Is:
POST GAME

Fat	Carb	Pro
27%	57%	16%
6g	28g	8g

Calories
196

**1 Serving
Equals**
½ Protein
1½ Grains
¼ Fruit
1 Fat

**If You Add
These Foods:**
0-½ Protein
2 Grains
2 Vegetables
1 Dairy
1 Fruit

OK To Use For:
PREGAME 2-3 HRS

POST GAME

As Is:

POST GAME

Fat	Carb	Pro
21%	57%	22%
3g	17g	6g

Calories
119

1 Serving Equals
½ Protein
1 Grain

___

If You Add These Foods:
2 Fruits

OK To Use For:

PREGAME 1-2 HRS

POST GAME

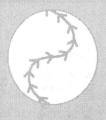

Two-on-Two Tuna Spread

1 can, 6 oz, water packed white tuna, drained
1 tablespoon fresh lemon juice
8 oz fat-free cream cheese, room temperature
2 tablespoons dry grated onion or onion flakes
½ teaspoon salt
1 teaspoon liquid smoke
1 serving low fat crackers or bagel chips

Mix above ingredients together in a bowl until well blended. Spread 2 tablespoons of the tuna mixture on your favorite low fat crackers or bagel chips (use 1 serving size of crackers or bagel chips as listed on box or package). Keep uneaten portion of tuna mixture covered and refrigerated.

Makes 1½ cups, 12 servings; serving size 2 tablespoons

Salmon Spread
Substitute 1 can of pink salmon, water packed. Be careful to remove any bones.

Chunky Salsa Chip Shot

1 cup store bought salsa
8 oz fat-free cream cheese,
    room temperature
3 tablespoons fat-free cheddar cheese,
    grated
36 Baked Tostitos Chips

Blend salsa and cream cheese together.
Sprinkle with cheddar cheese. Serve
with Baked Tostitos Chips.

Serves 3; serving size ⅓ of spread
and 12 chips

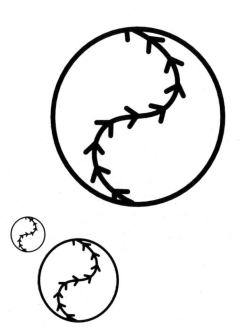

As Is:
Too High
in Protein
for Pre or
Post-Game

Fat	Carb	Pro
9%	61%	30%
2g	32g	16g

Calories
209

**1 Serving
Equals**
1½ Proteins
2 Grains
1 Vegetable

**If You Add
These Foods:**
1 Grains
½ Vegetable
3 Fruits

OK To Use For:

PREGAME 2-3 HRS

POST GAME

165

As Is:

PREGAME 1-2 HRS

POST GAME

Fat Carb Pro
6%   77%   17%
2g   46g   10g

Calories
237

1 Serving Equals
½ Protein
2 Grains
2 Fruits

If You Add These Foods:
½ Protein
2 Grains
2-2½ Vegetables
0-½ Fat

OK To Use For:

PREGAME 2-3 HRS

POST GAME

Ace Cinnamon Spread

4 oz fat-free cream cheese,
    room temperature
Cinnamon or pumpkin pie spice to taste
    (start with 1 teaspoon and go from
    there)
¼ cup dried cranberries or raisins or
    dried mixed fruit
2 large bagels (4 oz bagels), or
4 English muffins, or 8 slices of bread

Mix cream cheese, spices and dried
fruit together. Spread 2 tablespoons
of mixture on bread of choice.

Serves 4; serving size ½ bagel, or 1
English muffin or 2 slices of bread

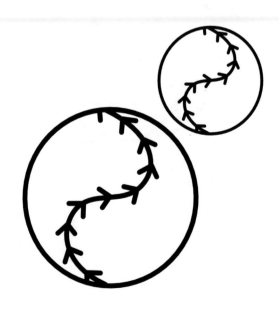

Fruit Be Forehand

½ cup spreadable fruit spread,
   your child's favorite flavor
3 oz fat-free cream cheese
6 slices whole wheat bread, or
   1½ large bagels (4 oz bagels), toasted

Mix fruit spread and cream cheese
together in a small bowl and spread on
bread or bagel, or spread fruit spread
on one slice of bread and cream cheese
on the other slice of bread. Keep unused
spread covered and refrigerated.

Serves 3; serving size 2 pieces of bread
or ½ bagel

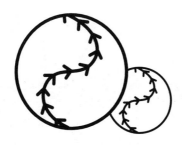

Fat	Carb	Pro
9%	77%	14%
3g	55g	10g

Calories
276

1 Serving
Equals
½ Protein
2½ Grains

If You Add
These Foods:
½ Protein
2 Grains
2 Vegetables
1 Dairy
2½ Fruits
1 Fat

OK To Use For:

PREGAME 3-4 HRS

POST GAME

Coach Eda's Winning Whipped Delight

½ cup fat-free whipped topping, room temperature

1 tablespoon reduced sugar orange marmalade preserves

2 cups washed and freshly sliced fruit (serve your child's favorites or mix and match strawberries, bananas, grapes, peaches, nectarines, kiwi, melon, blueberries or any other seasonal fruit)

By hand, mix marmalade and whipped topping, until blended. Serve fruit in individual bowls, spoon 2 teaspoons of topping on each serving. Refrigerate any unused topping in a covered container for up to two days.

Serves 3; serving size ⅔ cup

Tip
If marmalade is not a favorite in your home, use any reduced sugar fruit preserves instead. Experiment with different combinations of flavors. Let the kids do the mixing and matching.

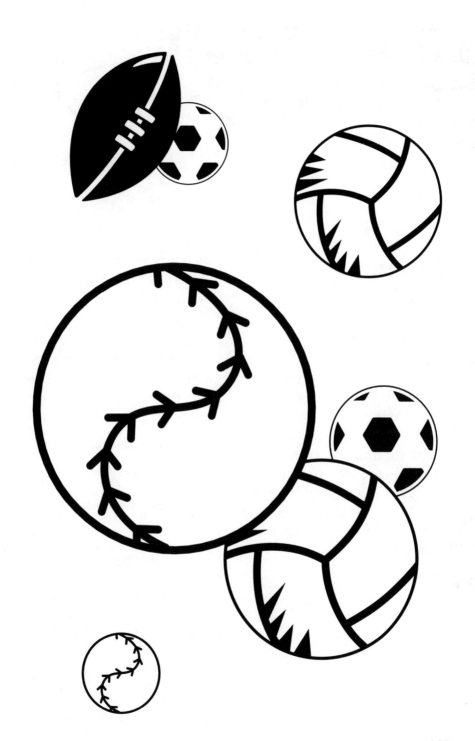

Additional Resources

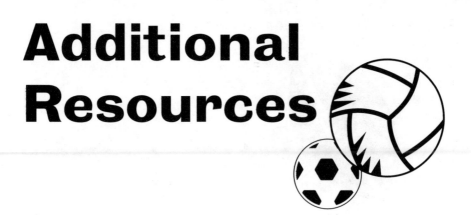

Conversion Formula

**Grams To Calories/
Calories To Grams**

For those who would like to do their own calculations:
Using the Food Label found on all food products, follow these instructions to determine a food's fat, carbohydrate, and protein percentages and how many calories are coming from each nutrient.

Nutrition Facts

Serving Size (28g)
Servings Per Container

Amount Per Serving

Calories 134   Calories from Fat 60

	% Daily Value*
Total Fat 6g	**9%**
Saturated Fat 2.5g	**14%**
Cholesterol 0mg	**0%**
Sodium 70mg	**3%**
Total Carbohydrate 18g	**6%**
Dietary Fiber 2g	**6%**
Sugar 15g	
Protein 2g	

Vitamin A 0%   •   Vitamin C 0%

Calcium 2%   •   Iron 4%

* Percent Daily Values are based on a 2,000 calorie diet. Your daily values may be higher or lower depending on your calorie needs.

	Calories:	2,000	2,500
Total fat	Less than	65g	80g
Saturated Fat	Less than	20 g	25g
Cholesterol	Less than	300mg	300mg
Sodium	Less than	2,400mg	2,400mg
Total carbohydrate		300g	375g
Dietary Fiber		25g	30g

Calories per gram
    Fat 9 • Carbohydrate 4 • Protein 4

**Sample Food Label:
Nut and Raisin Granola Bar**

Step 1: Values You Need To Know
- 1 gram of Fat = 9 calories
- 1 gram of Carbohydrates = 4 calories
- 1 gram of Protein = 4 calories

Step 2: Find Nutrition Values on the Food Label
Example...A Nut and Raisin Granola Bar has:
- 134 calories per serving
- 6 grams of Fat
- 18 grams of Carbohydrates
- 2 grams of Protein

Step 3: Calculation: (use values from Step 1)
- 6 grams of Fat x 9 calories per 1 gram of Fat =
  54 calories from Fat
- 18 grams of Carbohydrates x 4 calories per 1 gram of
  Carbohydrates = 72 calories from Carbohydrates
- 2 grams of Protein x 4 calories per 1 gram of Protein =
  8 calories from Protein

Step 4: To Find Percentage of Fats, Carbs, Protein:
Take the total from each category and then divide by the
total number of calories per serving.
- 54 calories from Fat divided by 134 calories =
  40% of the calories in the Granola Bar come from Fat
- 72 calories from Carbohydrates divided by 134 calories =
  54% of the calories come from Carbohydrates
- 8 calories from Protein divided by 134 calories =
  6% of the calories come from Protein

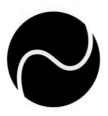

Books We Recommend

Play Hard, Eat Right: A Parent's Guide to Sports Nutrition for Children, By Debbie Sowell Jennings, Suzanne Nelson Steen, 1995, Chronimed Publishing, Minneapolis, MN

Good general nutrition and Sports Nutrition reference. It's a nice resource to have in your personal library.

Nancy Clark's Sports Nutrition Guidebook: Eating to Fuel Your Active Lifestyle, 2nd Edition, By Nancy Clark, 1997, Human Kinetics Publishers, Champaign, IL

Nancy Clark is a real pro, very well respected in the field of Sports Nutrition. Her books are easy to read, and provide good information about how to incorporate healthy nutrition practices into an active lifestyle.

Nutrition for Health, Fitness & Sport, 5th Edition, Melvin H. Williams, 1999, McGraw-Hill, Dubuque, IA

This book offers current research, practical activities and thorough coverage of the role nutrition can play in enhancing one's health, fitness and sports performance.

Nutrition for Sport & Exercise, 2nd Edition, Jacqueline R. Berning, Suzanne Nelson Steen, 1998, Aspen Publishers, Gaithersburg, MD

An in-depth resource for health professionals involved in the care of athletes. It was written by researchers in the field of Sports Nutrition. It's a good book for those who like their information delivered in great detail.

Newsletters and Websites

ACSM's Health and Fitness
www.Health-fitjrnl.com
800-486-5643

The American College of Sports Medicine publishes a journal called *Health & Fitness*. This journal is very easy to read and covers a variety of health topics such as ways to improve your overall diet, exercising methods, the latest health and fitness news, and all sorts of general information you'll find interesting and applicable.

Nutrition Action Healthletter
www.cspinet.org
202-332-9110

A product of the Center For Science in the Public Interest, the *Nutrition Action Healthletter* is straight to the point. It seeks to promote health through educating the public about nutrition and alcohol. It also provides information on how to become politically active on specific health issues. Visit the website for more information or to subscribe.

Gatorade Sports Institute's Sports Science Center
www.gssiweb.com
800-616-4774

This website covers a wide variety of Sports Medicine topics. It's a great resource for coaches and parents who want to keep up with the very latest research in the field of Sports Nutrition.

Sports Nutrition To Go!
www.SportsNutritionToGo.com

This is our website. See page 179 of this book for more information about us.

Give the Gift of "Great Snacks"

To Your Friends, Family, Colleagues, and Coaches

Order Additional Copies of
The Official Snack Guide For Beleaguered Sports Parents

1. To Place a Credit Card Order, Online
- Go to SportsNutritionToGo.com
- Click on The Sports Nutrition To Go! Logo
- Then Click on The OFFICIAL SNACK GUIDE page and follow ordering instructions

2. To Place a Credit Card Order, By Phone
Call (513) 321-7202 or use our Toll-Free number, 1-866-GO SNACK

3. To Order By Mail, Using a Check, or Credit Card
Copy and fill out this Order Form. Mail, along with your check or credit card information, to: WellCentered, Inc., 3414 Edwards Rd., Cincinnati, OH, 45208, ATT: Official Snack Guide

Please include a $4.75 shipping and handling fee for the first book you purchase. Add an additional $1.00 for each additional book ordered. Ohio residents, please include $1.00 sales tax, per book. (Canadian orders must include a Postal Money Order in U.S. Funds.) Please allow 15 days for delivery.

The Official Snack Guide
for Beleaguered Sports Parents
Order Form

_____

Name

_____

Address

_____

City   State   Zip

Please include a phone number or email address
(just in case we need to contact you to fulfill your order)

_____

Phone #

_____

email

❏ Payment By Check
❏ Payment By Credit Card [____Visa ____MasterCard ____Discover]

_____

Credit Card Number

_____

Expiration Date

_____

Signature

Number of Books _____ X $16.95 = $_____
Ohio Residents Only, Add Tax $1.00 per book $_____
Plus Shipping & Handling $4.75 for one book
(plus $1.00 for each additional book) $_____

Total Enclosed $_____

How To Contact The Authors

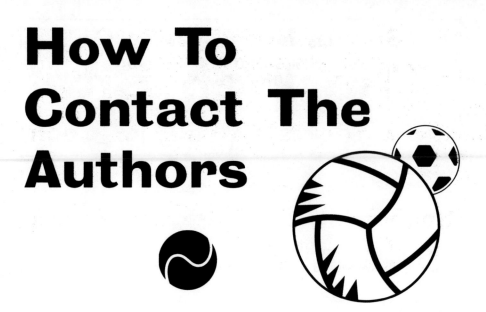

Dawn Weatherwax, RD, LD, ATC/L, CSCS, Sports Nutrition To Go!
Rita Nader Heikenfeld, CCP
Joan MacEachen Manzo, RN, BSN
Ellen Shuman, Executive Director, WellCentered, Inc.

Sports Nutrition To Go!
(513) 321-7202
(513) 533-7252 Fax
WellCentered, Inc.
3414 Edwards Rd.
Cincinnati, OH 45208

info@SportsNutritionToGo.com

Other WellCentered Books

Coming Soon!

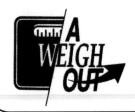

The A WEIGH OUT Workbook
An End To Diets and Out-of-Control Eating

The A WEIGH OUT Program specializes in working with people who are "Emotional Eaters". Emotional Eaters are people who eat when they are stressed, or bored, or lonely, etc...they use food, to varying degrees, to manage their moods. (Dietary changes, alone, will not fix that!)

For more information about A WEIGH OUT Programs and Services, the upcoming Workbook, Telephone and In-Person Coaching Services, TeleClasses, or Psychotherapy (Psychotherapy offered in-person in Greater Cincinnati only)

Please visit www.aweighout.com
Be sure to take the "Emotional Eating" Self-Test
on the Home Page!

Recipe Index

Brownies/Cookies
Annamarie's Major League Lemon Squares, 148
Championship Chocolate Cherry Brownies, 123
Cherry Pecan Power Bars, 124
Final Four Fruit Cocktail Cookies, 128
Home Run Chocolate Chippers, 129
Honey Bee-Line Cookies, 130
Over-The-Limit Oatmeal Treats, 126
Overtime Chocolate Chip Meringue Cookies, 132

Cakes
M.C.s Blueberry Break Coffee Cake,106

Dips/Spreads
(for fruits, chips, sandwiches, vegetables...)
Ace Cinnamon Spread, 166
All Star Apple-Raisin Breakfast Sandwich, 97
Backcourt Bagel Bites, 163
Cheddar Cheese Tofu Touchdown, 160
Chunky Salsa Chip Shot, 165
Coach Eda's Winning Whipped Delight, 168
Free Style Herb Spread, 156
Fruit Be Forehand, 167
Nutty Break-Away Graham Crackers, 159
Peanut Butter Crunch Break, 155
Rice Cake Rush, 161
Superbowl Veggies and Dip, 162
Two-on-Two Tuna Spread, 164

Drinks/Smoothies

Banana Honey Hat Trick, 82
Berry Banana Blitz, 81
Fast Break Cantaloupe Shake, 88
First Down Fruit & Soy Smoothie, 89
Half-Time Hot Chocolate, 111
Match Point Milk Shake & Malt, 83
Multi-Fruit Marathon, 90
Open-Ice Orange Creamsicle, 91
Peach Berry Bank Shot, 93
Ron's Pineapple Power Pitch, 87
Slam Dunk Chocolate Soy Shake, 84
Slap Shot Banana Smoothie, 86
Strawberry Banana Soy Sensation, 92
Triple Play Chocolate-Almond-Marshmallow Madness, 85

Egg Dishes

Eggs-treme Cheese Burrito, 110
Five-Minute Free Agent Omelet, 108

Frozen Treats

Base Hit Banana Popsicles, 150
Bella's Chocolate Rebound Bars, 135
Old-Timer's Orange Cubes, 149
Peanut Butter Puck Ice Cream Sandwiches, 152
Pink Lemonade Dream Team-Sicles, 151

Fruits

Home Court Chunky Applesauce, 146
Sideline Sun-Cooked Fruit Leather, 144
Sudden Death Chocolate Fruit Tips, 138

Muffins/Quick Breads
Banana Kick Bread, 104
Banana Wheat Germ MVP Muffins, 100
Freestyle Cinnamon Apple Oat Bran Muffins, 103
Granola-Almond Marching Muffins, 102

Pancakes/Waffles
Apple Pancake Power Play, 95
Center Court Waffles with Dribble Toppings, 98
Offside Oatmeal Pancakes, 96

Puddings/Parfaits
Chocolate Mousse Pudding Play, 136
Hole-In-One Granola Parfaits, 141
Paige's Vanilla-Chocolate Chip Power Pudding, 140

Snack Mixes
Countdown Grand Slam Trail Mix, 117
Cross Country Trail Mix, 116
Goalie Granola, 118
Pop-Up Pizza Popcorn, 122
Semi-Pro Snack Mix, 115
Shane's Tip-Off Taco Munchies, 120
Shot Put Snack Mix, 114
Trish's Switch Hitter Snack Mix, 113

Tortillas
Drop Kick Deli Wrap, 158
Volley Veggie Wrap, 157

Yogurt
Mary's Home Plate Yogurt, 142